start here

Breastfeeding and Infant Care
With Humor and Common Sense

Kathleen F. McCue, MS, RN, FNP-BC, IBCLC

Start Here:
Breastfeeding and Infant Care
With Humor and Common Sense

Kathleen F. McCue, MS, RN, FNP-BC, IBCLC

Illustrations by Erin McCue

Praeclarus Press, LLC
2504 Sweetgum Lane
Amarillo, Texas 79124 USA
806-367-9950
www.PraeclarusPress.com

DISCLAIMER
The information contained in this publication is advisory only and is not intended to replace sound clinical judgment or individualized patient care. The author disclaims all warranties, whether expressed or implied, including any warranty as the quality, accuracy, safety, or suitability of this information for any particular purpose.

ISBN: 978-1-946665-06-5

To my children, Adam and Erin, who taught me the true meaning of a mother's love.

acknowledgements

I am indebted to Dr. Kathleen Kendall-Tackett for her thoughtful guidance, good judgment, and unfailing support. I also express my appreciation to Janet Rourke, Alicia Ingram and the entire team at Hale Publishing.

Profound gratitude is due to my daughter Erin for her beautiful illustrations and her willingness to accept any art assignment. I am eternally grateful for my son's humor, which always sustains my soul no matter what I'm doing, and who gave me a lift when I needed it.

Deepest thanks to my mother, Ellen Kuhnen, who has worked endlessly at supporting my private lactation practice and has always tried to be there for me with her wisdom and insight.

I am indebted to my friend, Liat Katz, for her many helpful thoughts and suggestions, and for picking up the ball when I was running out of steam.

I learned what I know from all the parents who allowed me into their lives during very intimate times. I extend special thanks to all those mothers who worked tirelessly (ok, they were very tired) to find ways to implement my suggestions, but who also taught me that every mother-child relationship is unique. There were supportive fathers willing to get their hands dirty, and, of course, the sweet babies who made it all worth it, and then some. Their trials and tribulations have inspired me to put my thoughts and experiences into organized words.

A big debt of gratitude to the physicians at Children First Pediatrics (Cindy Fishman, Stuart Weich, Michael Datch, Jeannine Mogavero, Robin Chernoff, Liza Burns, Stacy Stryer, Kristen Dorsey, Erica Rupar, and Paul Porras), office manager (Rachel Bakersmith - my yes person), and their incredible nursing and support staff. My colleagues took me into their practice having total faith in my skills and abilities, and they embraced having a lactation consultant on staff.

Finally, in addition to those already mentioned, a special thank you to Dr. Reva Snow, who was there at the beginning and was a great resource for me.

Table of Contents

The newborn period can be an exciting one, but can leave most parents unsure of themselves. Most parents want to do everything they can to ensure their baby has the best chance of having a great life. After reading all the books, talking to all the friends, and eating all the right foods, they quickly learn, however, that taking care of their baby is not formulaic. Even taking classes does not adequately prepare new parents. (Taking a breastfeeding class without a baby is like taking a knitting class without needles and a ball of wool.) New parents search out answers to try to find their way. They ask everybody, and everybody seems to have a different answer, indicating that they know the best way to take care of a baby. This is the good news, however, because it means there's no ONE right way to do it. You should, therefore, take everybody's advice (including mine), stir it up in a big pot, and pull out the pieces that work for you and your baby. You should know, too, that you already have all the tools you need to do this parenting thing, and to do it well.

Rest assured, no matter what you do, you will discover there was a different way to do it that might have been better; I call this the learning curve. This reminds me of the story of the woman who raised her daughter, promising to do everything completely different than her mother did with her. Consequently, she raised a child just like her mother. If it takes you awhile to get the irony in this story, you're already tired.

So, if there are so many opinions and no one right way to parent, how do new parents know where to start? Over the past 37 years of practice, I've learned that lactation consulting is a careful balance of giving opinions, citing research, supporting, listening to, and learning from infants and their parents. A lot of lactation consulting has little to do with lactation and a lot to do with reassuring and providing parents with general hints at parenting newborns. As an experienced clinician, I generally know what works. Although in the land of babies and mothers, research is bringing more wonderful information to light, so methods and information we use as lactation consultants are changing with the times. I will impart my experience and some recent research, in hopes of helping you find some solid ground to build on.

Reviewing recent research on lactation consulting has allowed me to make my own clinical practice more accessible. This research and the new insights have helped me realize that everything we did in the past, like teaching breastfeeding classes with dolls to learn proper positioning (Mohrbacher, 2010), is passé. Instead, I learned that when we give very precise instructions to new moms, it can be overwhelming. The information can actually take the focus off the baby and put it on the instructions (Mohrbacher, 2010). When moms pay more attention to a set of written instructions than to their newborns, it's never a good thing. That's why this book is decidedly not a "How-to" book. You can find many books like that on breastfeeding. Rather, this is a book of thoughts and suggestions on breastfeeding and baby care, created in the hope that you might find some helpful information and incorporate it into what you already know, to create a repertoire that works for you.

In reading the 2010 research on best practices, I knew I had to make changes in the way I thought about breastfeeding and in the way I practiced lactation consulting. I was overwhelmed with making a paradigm shift until one day a nest of baby birds appeared on my front porch flower wreath. The mother bird on my door is responsible for helping me understand how best to help you. Day after day, rain or shine, I watched the mother and marveled at how her instincts prevailed. I wondered how she seemed to know exactly what to do, and when to do it. Who taught her how to build this perfect nest? Then I realized that she tapped into her instincts. Period. That's exactly what you need to do to be successful; you need to tap into that inborn hard-wiring that we, as lactation consultants and healthcare professionals, have only begun to understand. You already have the basic instincts you need; all you have to do is trust them.

Breastfeeding can be compared to falling in love; it's not a thinking thing. It's something that evolves and takes on a life of its own. Too often, in our quest for knowledge, we try to intellectualize breastfeeding and make it an activity that is a learned skill. We look for the "right way" to do it. Low and behold, there IS no right way, there's your way and your baby's way. Much like a romantic couple finds their way in the world, you and your baby will find your way to successful breastfeeding if you just trust your instincts. Nature helps us and our babies prepare for that.

The first 40 days of your child's life are the most important in terms of laying down your structure, maximizing your milk supply, and basically getting the hang of it all. This book is designed to provide you with hints on how to do all this and remind you that you already have the knowledge, strength, and skills to be a successful parent. On a personal note, I believe that having a sense of humor is imperative in this endeavor.

Note: In this book, I refer to moms as she/her and babies as he/him. I realize that babies come in both genders. But sometimes the sentences get confusing if you refer to both mom and baby as she/her.

I Can't Read Now, My Baby's Crying!

First things first - if your baby is hysterically CRYING as you read this, (until you read more information on feeding cues) interpret this as HUNGER and FEED. If you're breastfeeding, it's time to get the breast out. You can go straight to the next section on latching if necessary. If you're reading this book because breastfeeding doesn't seem to be working for you, then read the next two paragraphs.

As a desperate measure, you may need to give your baby a tiny bit of formula right now. I know, I know, this is the beginning of a book on breastfeeding AND a lactation consultant is writing it, but there are some situations that warrant giving your baby formula right now, even if you are committed to breastfeeding. If your baby has had a 7-10% weight loss or more, few wet diapers, and a weak cry, I believe that formula can be a very temporary stopgap measure to get you through an hour or two of reading and should not permanently damage the breastfeeding relationship. I call this safeguarding breastfeeding. Well-nourished babies do a better job of breastfeeding. This is NOT an endorsement of artificial breastmilk; this is a veto against hunger.

As I just said, there are circumstances prior to primary engorgement (your milk coming in) and beyond, when it's simply medically necessary to use a bit of formula. These circumstances will be discussed in later chapters. Keep the amount to about an ounce or less if it's during the first week, and use a quality orthodontic nipple, preferably slow flow. If the baby is still crying after the ounce, then latch the baby to the breast and/or provide lots of skin-to-skin contact. You'll see a difference pretty quickly as the baby's hands, which were previously clenched, will probably look more relaxed and open, like a flower blooming. Now that you have some quiet time, start reading with baby on you, skin-to-skin.

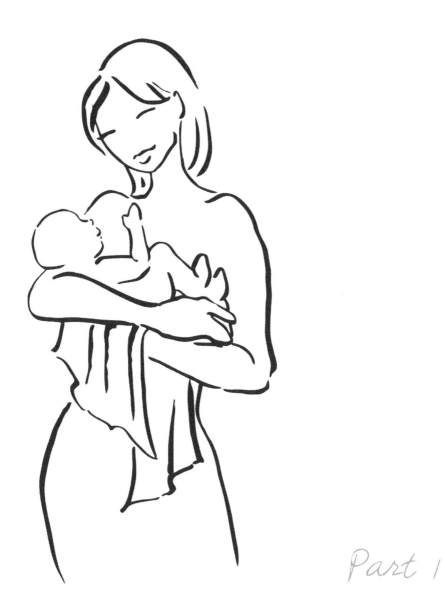

Part 1

BREASTFEEDING OR NOT, HERE I COME

Chapter 1

Feeding

"You need to be a warrior!" These were the words I had one mother tell me she wished someone had said to her when she made the decision to breastfeed. She said that if she knew it was going to be this difficult, she would have mentally prepared herself. Although it's not usually "this difficult," you should work on your warrior skills. By this, I mean you should become tenacious with breastfeeding and patient with yourself and your baby. You will find your way...there are lots of paths.

You and Your Breasts Need Support! (And I'm Not Talking About a Bra)...Your Partner

You've decided to breastfeed. You've been walking around with breasts on your chest since you were about 12; now it's time to use them. You've read the books on breastfeeding, your breasts have grown (and grown and grown), you have bought breastfeeding pumps, pads, creams, and pillows, and you feel ready. The fact is, though, that although you may have the equipment and may be physically ready to breastfeed, you also need to have the psychological and social support for breastfeeding. Your partner, and perhaps family, needs to be ready, too. You will be more successful at breastfeeding (being able to do it longer and more exclusively) if you feel confident in what you are doing. We are always more confident in what we are doing when we feel supported and helped with our decisions—and breastfeeding is no exception. Without support from those around you, you may feel burdened by breastfeeding because you feel isolated and overwhelmed.

Your partner can be involved in breastfeeding in many different ways. First, it is important that you have conversations with him or her during pregnancy about your thoughts and expectations about breastfeeding. If your partner is made to feel meaningfully involved early on, then breastfeeding can be incorporated as a positive part of your growing family's lifestyle. As you discuss the benefits of breastfeeding together, the realization might become clear of the (sometimes sacrificial) gift that you are giving to your baby and to your family. Your partner can start helping by attending a breastfeeding class with you or researching lactation resources that are available should you need help after the baby arrives. After the baby arrives, your partner can continue to be supportive by taking care of household and baby chores—such as diaper changing and cooking, so you do not feel overwhelmed. Also, your mate can take care of the baby while you do things to take care of yourself, like showering or eating. This helps your partner build a bond with the baby that you already have by breastfeeding. Your partner can also bring the baby to you for overnight feedings.

Your Extended Family and Friends

"Why do grandparents and grandchildren get along so well? They have the same enemy—the mother."-- Claudette Colbert (Top 25 Grandparent Quotations, 2010)

Social support is necessary for the breastfeeding relationship because your relationship with your child does not exist in a vacuum—you are part of a broader community that influences how you feel and act about breastfeeding. While your partner is part of your everyday life, you have others in your community that may influence your breastfeeding experience. People in your life will share with you their views about breastfeeding, and often provide unsolicited advice on how good a job they think you are doing at breastfeeding. In order not to take their negativity too much to heart, it is important to understand where their views or comments may be coming from. Your parents or grandparents may not understand your choice to breastfeed or your choice to breastfeed long-term because breastfeeding was not always accepted or in-style when they were raising you or their children. Men in your life may shy away from wanting to talk about or witness breastfeeding because they view breasts only as sexual objects. It's also a possibility that they just have never had any experience with breastfeeding babies or mothers. In the beginning, motherhood is such a sensitive time because of the tremendous hormonal and lifestyle changes that you are going through. Negative comments can be extremely hurtful at this time, and it is up to you to remain strong in your convictions—in breastfeeding and in parenting—even with any negativity you might experience. For some women, successful breastfeeding is successful mothering, and when those around you question your skills at breastfeeding, it can strike you right in your gut. When a well-intentioned grandmother tells you that your milk is "no good," you can help her understand how important it is for you to feel supported and how much her negativity can end up interfering with your decision to breastfeed.

There's no such thing as bad milk. Many well-meaning friends and family members will sabotage a mother's decision simply by saying the baby is still hungry right after you feed her. They all need to back off, plain and simple. I actually had a mom tell me that a nurse in the hospital told her that her baby was crying because he wanted a hamburger and all she had was a French fry. That's just plain mean. Remember that, especially during the first week, your milk supply is getting established. And, although you can value your relationship with specific people, you do not have to take all of their advice on parenting or breastfeeding. This is especially true with your mother. It is so easy for your own mother to "push your buttons" BECAUSE she installed them. Even though others may have more experience with breastfeeding or parenting, YOU are the mother now, so tap into those maternal instincts and have confidence in making decisions for yourself and your baby. Now is the time to decide if you are the baby of the mother or the mother of the baby.

After Delivery—OK, Baby's Here, Now What?

There's a golden window during the first two hours after birth where babies will be fairly awake and nurse well. For the next 22 hours, it may be more difficult to arouse him. Try hand expressing some colostrum onto your nipple (described later in the book) and bringing baby up to the breast (even if all you get is a lick and a few minutes of suckling). Express (squeeze) until you see golden liquid coming from the small openings in the nipple. The labor and delivery nurse might be able to assist you with this. The bottom line is, the more your baby stays on you, with you, and next to you, the better the breastfeeding and bonding will go.

In an ideal world, you deliver the baby, and he is immediately put to the breast for about an hour. The baby is THEN taken away for weighing, measuring, foot printing, etc. and returned back to the breast/chest for more skin-to-skin for the remainder of the second hour. For the rest of the day, you keep your baby with you while you recover from the birth!

On the second day, the baby is brought to you to breastfeed frequently, and you continue to keep him skin-to-skin. Don't expect a perfect breastfeeder (you or him). Talk to him frequently, look into his eyes, and start to learn as much as you can about your new baby. Some babies will already be doing a beautiful job of breastfeeding and others will still be learning, it's all normal and to be expected.

Try to keep the baby "rooming-in" with you during any nights if possible. Rooming-in allows you and your baby to form an early attachment that will benefit both of you. Physiologically, the baby will learn from you at this stage how his body works—he will adjust his breathing, heart rate, and temperature appropriately, instead of being distracted by the lights and noise of a nursery. Rooming-in will also benefit your body, which will learn to produce lots of milk as it learns what the baby next to you wants.

Early and frequent skin-to-skin contact has profound psychological and neurological effects on you and your baby—allowing for early attachment and bonding that will make the baby feel safe, promote early brain development, and allow you to cue in to your baby's needs. Rooming-in may actually help you sleep more—you might sleep deeper and longer in the hospital knowing your baby is safely lying right next to you and not away from you with someone else.

Please don't let the nurses whisk your baby away and feed him a bottle in the nursery. I know you're tired, I know you might be in some pain. At a bare minimum, if you really feel it will help you, let them keep him, but have them bring him to you whenever he cries.

The positive trend toward rooming-in is somewhat of a newer phenomenon. When my son Adam was born, they brought him to me in the middle of the night. He was very cold and the nurses told me that the isolette (baby warmer) broke. They apologized, asking me to keep him next to my body to increase his temperature. After an hour, they took him back and told me not to worry because they had turned the "temperature up as high as they could." They were sure he'd be "nice and warm now." After they took him, I lay there...and all I could think about was how they were going to ROAST my new baby. Since they wouldn't let me have him back, I got up, dragged myself down the hall, and sat next to the isolette until the next morning. I sure wish it were 2010 and someone would have simply suggested skin-to-skin contact for the entire night. That's all it would have taken to regulate his temperature and for me to get a good night's sleep.

Stay Right and You'll Never Go Wrong

There's a beautiful phenomenon that happens as a result of you and your baby coming together. Generally, when we think and act, we use both sides of our brain. However, certain types of thinking are more strongly associated with the right or the left side of the brain. We know that the right brain is our touchy-feely, intuitive, emotional side and our left brain is our logical, rational, and analytical side. Babies are always right-brained because they haven't learned to cognitively THINK yet.

Current research suggests that we synchronize our brains with our babies, making our right brain more active and dominant than our left brain after we give birth (Mohrbacher, 2010). This synchronization allows us to become further in touch with our newborns, and it explains so much! It's the reason we have a difficult time following instructions and keeping track of things in the early weeks (Eidelman, Hoffmann, & Kaitz, 1993). I wish I would have known this in MY early postpartum days. I jokingly used to say that the baby was taking all my brain cells as an excuse for my fumblings. So, when we MATCH our babies more, we become in sync with them.

Sometimes, we are not synchronized with our babies because we rely too heavily on the left side of our brain. It is interesting to note that, "unlike other mammals, a human mother can use her intellect to overrule her innate behaviors and emotions" (Mohrbacher, 2010, p. 37). This means we can over-think mothering, nurturing, and breastfeeding. In my clinical experience, the smarter and more educated a mom is, the more she tries to use her intellect to learn how to breastfeed. This makes sense for a woman who has used that same intellect to get her where she is in life, but it just doesn't always bode well for breastfeeding. Becoming a new mom and progressing through breastfeeding can be challenging for any woman, no matter what her walk in life.

Time to Feed--Everyone Comfortable and

in Position?

In order to ensure success with breastfeeding, you need to be kind to yourself in the beginning, and give yourself some time to really get into this new rhythm of your life. Successful breastfeeding comes when your baby eats adequately when he's hungry, and you and your baby are comfortable while you are feeding him. This is easier said than done, but it becomes easier with a bit of experience. I will provide some hints to get started.

Being Kind to Yourself

In my experience, most mothers, especially first-time mothers, are not adequately prepared for the amount of time and energy a new baby takes. There are several reasons for this struggle during the first couple months. I believe the primary reason is the mothers' lack of good, solid stretches of uninterrupted sleep. I've often compared nursing mothers to soldiers in foxholes, meaning they always have to maintain some degree of vigilance 24/7, never letting their guard down. They're listening to every sound their newborn makes, even heavy breathing. They're vigilant for signs of discomfort and feeding cues. I believe this can zap a mom's energy. Of course, there are other reasons for mothers feeling overwhelmed: hormonal shifts, physical discomfort (either from episiotomies, swollen breasts, hemorrhoids, or sutures), and too many well-meaning visitors.

In general, mothers often become overwhelmed because they tend to think they should naturally be able to do this mother/baby thing, without any direction, preparation, or outside help. You may feel like you're being graded on this, so-to-speak, and that the job you're doing is a direct reflection on how "good" a mother you are in the eyes of others. There are many ways to parent successfully and to breastfeed successfully, and there is no shame in getting help to find your way and help tap into your instincts. There are plenty of resources available once you feel comfortable reaching out. You can start by talking with people in your support system, your OB/GYN or midwife, a lactation consultant, or your child's healthcare practitioner.

With all that in mind, give yourself some credit for all that you are going through. Remember that babies naturally love everything about their mothers--their faces, their voices, their smell, and the feel of their bodies when skin-to-skin. Be confident that you will build upon your baby's natural love for you by developing a breastfeeding relationship that will become easier and more enjoyable; it just might take a bit of time and patience.

Getting Into Your Rhythm

How often should you feed your baby? How long? Which breast and how long on each side? Should you be waking to feed? These are all rhythm questions, and ones that are best answered by you and your baby. It's like learning to dance. You might watch a dance and try to emulate it, but you'll put your own special signature on your moves. In dancing, sometimes partners are not always matching moves, and that's OK. After more dances, you'll begin to understand and anticipate each other's moves—that's what will make your dance unique.

Of course, there are many things that can interfere with your initial rhythm and throw the dance off a bit. These include medications used during labor, traumatic births (for mom and/or baby), jaundice (makes babies very sleepy), c-section deliveries, early separation of mother and baby (especially separation resulting in an inability to feed within the first hour or two), illness in either you or your baby, and no opportunity for lots of skin-to-skin contact in the immediate hours after birth.

So, what types of things encourage the best breastfeeding rhythms to develop? This list includes (Mohrbacher, 2010):

- Rooming-in
- Quiet, uninterrupted time with your baby
- Lots of skin-to-skin contact
- Avoidance of pacifiers
- Frequent feeds

Rooming-In and Quiet Uninterrupted Time With Your Baby

The benefits of rooming-in were discussed previously in this chapter and include mother and baby attuning to each other's needs, early bonding and attachment, and the opportunity for frequent and helpful skin-to-skin contact. These can also be accomplished at home when you ensure that you have quiet, comfortable, uninterrupted time with your baby.

Skin-to-Skin Contact

Because babies naturally love everything about their mothers, when moms couple skin-to-skin contact with TOUCHING, TALKING, and looking into baby's eyes, it helps a baby settle and stay calm. This contact helps you bond with your baby, helps your baby form an attachment to you, and actually allows you to release oxytocin, a hormone needed to breastfeed (Mohrbacher, 2010).

Frequent Feeds

Never try to get your baby onto a schedule in the early days. Feel free to feed, feed, feed— like you're fattening up the holiday goose (so to speak). Parents will say that their children hate being naked or cry so much they must have colic. I'm pretty sure they're just "hangry," as my daughter would say (combination of "hungry" and "angry"). When kids are well-fed, you should be able to lay them on a mound of snow in the yard, and they'll sleep calmly (not really, but you get the idea). It should look like fleet-week in New York. They should be out cold and sleep anywhere! If not, it's OK to keep feeding. If the baby overeats, he'll send it right back up in your direction...in that case, take note of how much he overfed, wait a half hour or so until you see feeding cues, and re-feed. The stomach is not perfect at emptying 100% of its contents, so there is still milk in there. Although this is rare, I wanted you to be prepared...just in case.

Frequent feeds are necessary because it is an instinctual and natural need of babies. When babies are in the womb, they're fed continuously. They have this wonderful umbilical cord that's sending nutrients down 24/7. So, it is no wonder why babies want to eat so frequently after they are born. Their stomachs are very small and, therefore, only hold about an ounce or so. Also, the amount of time and energy a newborn takes to feed is based on the fact that we're mammals, and our natural feeding patterns are pre-determined.

In essence, different species have different parameters for frequency of feeding based on how much protein and fat there is in their milk. Species fall into three categories: those who have intermittent contact with their mothers (mammals that are mature enough at birth to follow their moms around, like giraffes and cows), those that can be left in nests or burrow (like the deer and the rabbit), and those that have continuous contact with their mothers (meaning mammals that need to be held against their mother's body to stay warm and are carried constantly) (Mohrbacher, 2010). The milk of the "constant-carry mammals" (apes, marsupials, and humans) has the lowest levels of fat and protein, meaning that babies need to be fed pretty much around the clock (Mohrbacher, 2010). When we understand the reason for frequent feedings, it can make it all seem more natural and normal. Now you know why it is not reasonable for you to expect your baby to sleep for several hours at a time, throughout the day AND night, at least in the beginning.

Ensuring Baby Eats When Hungry

To ensure that your baby eats when he is hungry, it is important to learn to understand and read his cues for wanting to feed. When babies are hungry, they increase their activity level, put their hands to their mouths to suck them, and if you aren't paying attention, they'll start to cry. Crying is a late sign of hunger. Babies will also exhibit behaviors that indicate they are seeking their mother's breast. Because of a lack of understanding, some moms will interpret breast-seeking behaviors negatively. I've heard moms tell me they think their baby doesn't like them (or their breasts) because the baby tries to bat at the breast and push away. I always explain that babies will suck their hands, bat at the breast (to stimulate the nipple to stick out), and then latch on. Their arm movements shouldn't be interpreted negatively; it's a great survival instinct at work. Therefore, if you understand and can interpret what your baby is doing, you'll understand that this is all very natural and is helping baby to orient himself to the breast (Mohrbacher, 2010).

If you put a baby, tummy-side down, on mom's belly while she is lying down, he will innately find mom's breast (Widstrom et al., 1987). What babies do to get there varies, but it always utilizes their feet or hands and mouths to help them find and take the breast. They might put their hands in their mouths, open and close their fists, move their arms and legs around, lift their heads up, bob their heads, crawl, and/or step their feet down and push (Mohrbacher, 2010). Just watch them. It's amazing! Once they get to where they're going, to help transfer milk, they suck, move their jaws around, and swallow. Once their faces are into the breast, they find the breast and nipple by rooting (turning the head side to side with an open mouth) and feeling the breast on their chins (which causes the chin to drop down). They then stick their tongues out over their lower gums and begin to suckle (Genna, 2008). It is interesting to note that there are no differences in feeding behaviors whether babies are awake or asleep! Better them than us!

What are more innate cues you should look for that indicate your baby may be hungry and ready to feed? Yes, they involve the classic things you probably already know about, like rooting (looking for the breast), sucking, and swallowing, but there are lots more. So far, 20 have been identified that help babies get the breast, and, therefore, get the milk (Mohrbacher, 2010). Now before you get too excited, most babies will not use all reflexes at all feedings. That would just be exhausting. The best position for mom, the one that gets babies really going, is when mom is laid-back or semi-reclined, like the Romans, waiting for grapes. This position really makes nursing very simple in the early days. Researchers have suggested that when babies feed on their tummies, breastfeeding is much less of a struggle (Colson, 2008), and suggest that human newborns are meant to be tummy feeders... like puppies and hamsters (Mohrbacher, 2010).

I must note here that when I originally read that "tummy feeder" statement in one of my newest research books, I did NOT believe it. I set out to prove this theory incorrect, only to be proven dead wrong. I was duly amazed at how many of my mothers, not only marveled at how well their babies did in this position, but also commented positively on how much more rest and relaxation they got during these feeds! Just in case you're curious, I did receive many jaundiced looks from mom when I first suggested it. It did need to be sold as an idea worth trying before many brave souls climbed up onto the baby's exam table and bared both breasts and tummies for my book experiment.

OK, so how do we trigger babies to show us their breast-seeking behaviors? U.K. midwife and researcher, Suzanne Colson (2003), suggests that a mother hold her baby so that baby's face, neck, chest, tummy, and legs are closely wrapped around mom's body contour, offering unrestricted access to the breast. This means, we CUDDLE them…see? Natural instinct, right? Who doesn't want to cuddle their baby? You don't have to lie all the way back, just shift your hips forward and slouch. Also, foot rubbing will stimulate your baby to suck.

Your Comfort

Build a nest. I started this book talking about the mother bird on my front door wreath. Some of the same instincts that helped her build her nest should encourage you to build yours. By this, I mean you should find a special place at home that will make you feel happy and comfortable.

Many times, mothers will come to me to help them and ask me to just "check the latch." I always say that if the baby is gaining weight, transferring milk, and mom is happy, what's the point? (In other words, if it ain't broke, don't fix it). I will, however, help a mom who's having difficulty finding the right position for her and baby, and offer several suggestions. In doing so, I ask the mom to first show me her most comfortable position for watching TV. I then take it from there. She already knows what's comfortable. I just have to help her figure out how to incorporate her little one in next to her.

Baby's Comfort and Latch--Hey, Hold That Thing for Me, My Jaw Is Getting Tired Here!

Babies have a difficult time tilting their heads forward (with chin to the chest) to drink (Glover & Wiessinger, 2008). It makes sense, I mean, try to put YOUR chin to your chest and swallow…almost impossible! After babies take the breast deeply, they need to tilt their heads back slightly. That will actually help open the throat. Kind of like swallowing your prenatal vitamin, you have to put your head back a bit after your drink of water.

The Perfect Latch - Nine Tried-and-True Recommendations for Latching

1. You should latch a baby before they're showing feeding cues. This will mean that you engage in frequent feeding in the early days, which will also help with your primary engorgement.

2. Don't PUSH. We learned that as children…Allow your baby to take your breast at his own pace instead of pushing his head. Otherwise, you'll probably get pushed back and that's just not the point. Some will latch quickly, like a barracuda; others will slowly do you the favor of latching. It's all normal and, for some, may vary

from feed to feed. Keep in mind that it's almost impossible to latch a crying baby. First calm him down. Temporarily (a minute or less) swaddling can help in this instance (see Swaddling or Bundling section in this chapter).

3. It's best to try to latch a baby with a feeding difficulty to the breast when they're drowsy or asleep.

4. There is no need to vary positions for ANY reason unless you want to.

5. For all size breasts, it's best to keep the breast close to its natural height during breastfeeding. For moms who are large breasted, all they need to do is to keep the nipple and areola supported during a feed, which is a lot less work.

6. If your baby needs a little help taking the breast, sandwich it or shape it by squeezing it together, so it's easier for the baby to latch deeply. Make sure you squeeze it parallel (to match the same direction) to the baby's lips. For example, if you want to smush down a big sub sandwich to fit into your mouth, you wouldn't squeeze it left to right. You'd squeeze it down to fit into your mouth.

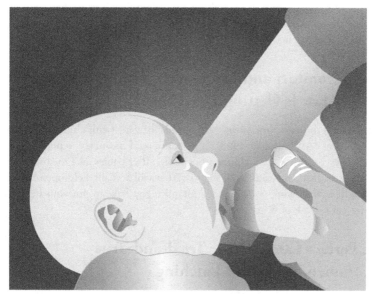

Figure 1.0 The Breast Sandwich

7. It's very helpful to have baby take the breast DEEPLY (I can't emphasize this point enough, it's key) because he actually draws the milk out by dropping his tongue and creating a vacuum (Geddes, Kent, Mitoulas, & Hartmann, 2008). This means your baby doesn't squeeze it out, rather he creates a vacuum and it squirts out. When the baby gets the nipple in the exact right spot in the mouth, it won't hurt or cause trauma to the breast because it is in a virtual "comfort zone" (Mohrbacher & Kendall-Tackett, 2010).

8. This is baby's job, too. No need for you to do all the work.

9. When you de-latch, always get your finger between your baby's gums, so he can't BITE down on the breast as you withdraw it. In other words, break the suction first!

Breastfeeding Positions

Positions are given as suggestions, much as you would find diagrams of stretches, postures, or exercises in a fitness book. Your own repertoire of favorite positions should not be limited to the ones below. However, augmented by these possibilities, you just might find one more comfortable for you or baby.

Tummy Feeding or the Reclining Position are both great choices for starting positions. These holds can be especially helpful if you've given birth in a hospital and will spend most of your time in bed. It's surprising how comfortable and easy these positions can be.

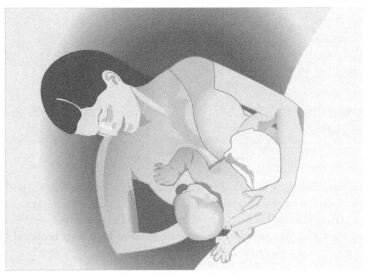

Figure 1.1 Tummy Feeding

The football hold can be another perfect starting hold for many reasons. First, you can see your baby's face and eyes very easily. Second, you can also see exactly what you're doing with your nipple/breast when you bring it to your baby's mouth. If you've had a c-section, there's also the benefit of not bearing weight on your tummy.

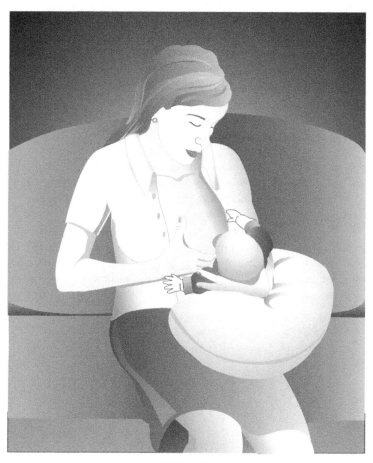

Figure 1.3 Football Hold

It can seem awkward at first, but it may become your favorite feeding position, so try it. It can be helpful to hold the breast in the C-Hold (meaning your fingers make a perfect C when holding your right breast and a perfect backward C when holding your left). You will use the opposite hand to hold your breast with the thumb on top. Let's start with the right breast.

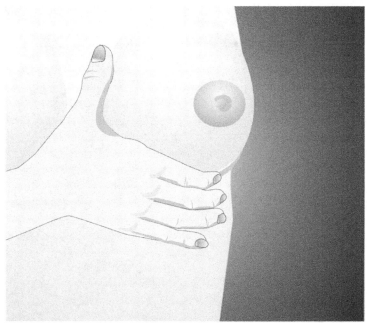

Figure 1.4 C-Hold

- Hold the right breast in the C-Hold with your left hand and have baby under your right arm, with the back of his neck in the comfortable part of your right hand.

- Bring your baby to your breast after you've expressed a drop or two of milk on the tip of your nipple, using breast compressions.

- Allow baby to take the breast at his own pace, although it's alright to gently help him latch. Be gentle and do not push the head. Rather, gently guide your baby. It can be helpful to have your nipple pointing up toward the ceiling (your left thumb can be smushing down over the areola a bit to accomplish this and to help make the breast sandwich), and feel the nipple brush past baby's upper lip. Don't be surprised if it takes a few attempts. Everyone is still in the learning phase.

A good, comfortable, but supportive, pillow under your baby can help you. Babies are born with two fears: loud noises and falling (both will cause a startle reflex where they jerk their arms open). If his head feels like a tennis ball on a two-by-four wood plank, he's not going to be able to concentrate on eating and hanging out at the breast. Think about how long you're willing to sit at a restaurant with uncomfortable chairs...uhhhhhhh "CHECK PLEASE!"

Here are some illustrations of some classic, tried and true breastfeeding positions.

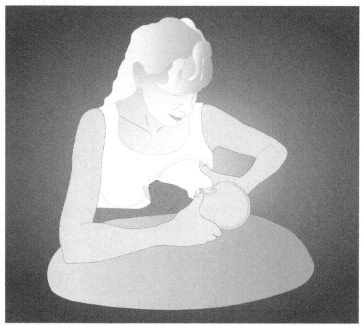

Figure 1.5 Cross Cradle Hold

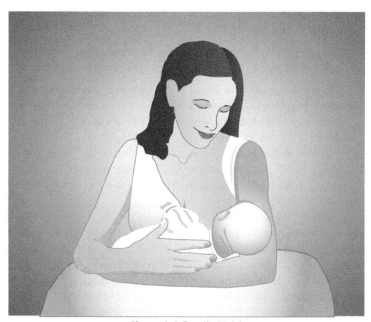

Figure 1.6 Cradle Hold

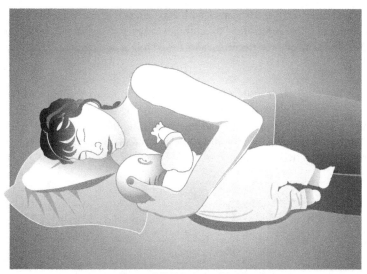

Figure 1.7 Side Lying Hold

With all upright positions, if you've used your fingers to guide the breast into your baby's mouth, remember to release your thumb upward (away from the breast) after your baby latches on. Otherwise, it may be like beavers building a dam in your breast. If you continue to make a thumb indentation print on the breast by squeezing in one place throughout the entire feed, you may end up with a plugged duct. From working with moms in my practice, I've found it works a little better if you use that thumb as a compressor (to squeeze the milk out and down) by moving it either up and down or moving it from the chest wall toward the nipple.

If easier or more comfortable, you may choose to keep your four fingers under the working breast to support it. When your baby is suckling in the football hold, he may be lifting a two to three pound breast with his chin. After a few sucks, it's simply not worth it. Suppose you had to lift up a weight every time you wanted a peanut. How long would you be able to or want to keep it up?

I remember asking a mom to try feeding her baby using the Madonna hold….. and she asked me how "Madonna" fed her baby? Mother of God or rock star? You decide.

Swaddling or Bundling: Bundle of Joy?

Swaddling can be great to help calm a baby and get him to sleep, but not so great to encourage their breast-seeking behaviors. Babies should be allowed to move about when possible. If babies are swaddled all the time, they don't wake as often, and, therefore, won't feed as much.

Swaddling after birth is associated with less competent early suckling and later establishment of breastfeeding. "Swaddling is associated with a greater weight loss, shorter duration of breastfeeding, and lower infant temperature" (Mohrbacher, 2010, p. 69).

On the flip side, when really necessary, and after a proper feeding and burping, it can be a great "off switch" and temporary calming technique. Just don't overdo it. Also, you'll want to keep in mind that swaddling for sleep increases the risk of SIDS (Sudden Infant Death Syndrome). Always remember to keep your baby on his back to sleep (Kemp, 2005).

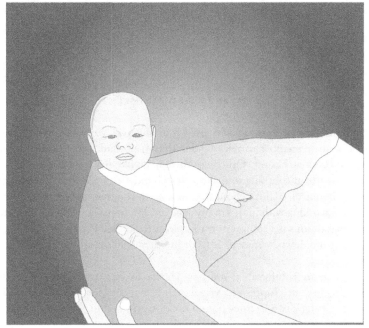

Figure 1.8 Swaddling 1

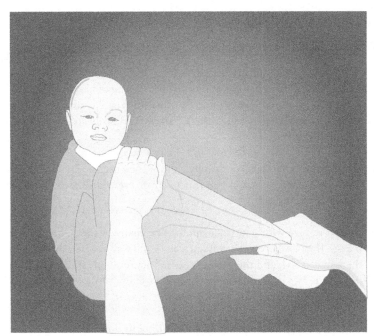
Figure 1.9 Swaddling 2

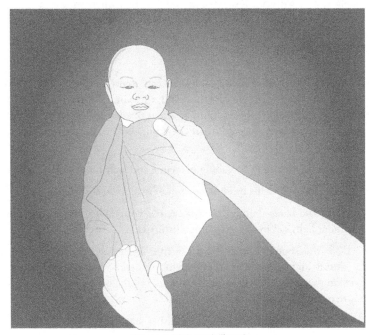
Figure 1.10 Swaddling 3

Understanding Your Baby's Sucking: Wall Stickers and Sleepy Slugs

Some kids suck so hard that when they breastfeed they're like land-sharks or barracudas, and their jaws are snapping even before mom's blouse is unbuttoned. One of the doctors in our practice jokes that these kids could "suck the chrome off a gear shift." I also call them "wall-stickers." They could easily attach to a wall with those lips and just stay there.

There are also the "gourmets" or "sleepy slugs." They use the "suck and snooze" method of dining. After a few meager sucks, their eyes roll into the back of the head for a much needed rest.

Infants are so in love with you (their mom) that many of them literally collapse at the breast. They love everything about you— the way you sound, the way you smell, the way you feel, and the way you taste. They're simply in heaven and don't even know you're two separate people, so, of course, they doze off! Life is so much less confusing when you're with the one you love, isn't it?

Unlike bottle feeding, breasts don't have a continuous flow for the entire feeding. Babies will start to nurse, and then after a burst of about 17-20 sucks, stop, flutter, and usually restart within a few seconds. It's just like when we eat and put our fork down for a minute, or pause mid-scoop into the mashed potatoes to finish our sentence. This is a normal eating pattern. Don't expect your baby to just keep sucking down milk without a short break.

If you're thinking the pause is too long, you can count to ten (if you insist), in seconds--one one thousand, two one thousand, three one thousand, etc. The wall-sticker will generally resume his vacuum attack at this point. If you get all the way up to 10 and baby is still out cold, there are a bunch of ways to stimulate him to restart his suck:

- Speak to your baby by calling his name and wait for a sucking reply.
- Rub the back of his head or bottom of his foot.
- With the hand holding the breast, use your index finger to come out under baby's chin and give him a little tickle.
- Rub the shoulder with a little gentle squeezing action between your thumb and index finger. (I'm convinced there's a hidden string under the skin that goes directly from the shoulder to the bottom of the baby's chin that this rubbing stimulates.)
- Start gentle breast compressions, either starting at your chest wall and smushing toward the nipple or just a gentle, solid squeeze mid-breast.

Whichever method you pick, you may prefer to stop when the baby starts to suck, so it becomes Pavlovian and the baby makes the connection... "Oh right, right, I'm supposed to be sucking here... I've got work to do." It's like getting a dirty look from your boss that almost automatically makes you start working again.

My rule is to never do anything mean to the baby or anything you would not like done to you. Parents have said that they've tried ice cold, wet washcloths on the baby's face or blowing in the baby's face to keep them feeding. Remember, if you wouldn't want it done to you, they probably don't want it done to them, either.

Additionally, you don't necessarily have to be rubbing the baby the whole time he's eating for any reason other than it feels right to you. For some babies, I have seen it be annoying or distracting. I believe constant rubbing is actually one of the ways moms deal with their *own* stress. How would you like it if somebody rubbed you the whole time you were eating your sandwich? "Hey, bug off! Get lost, lady. I'm eating my sandwich here!" Just another thought —it may or may not apply to all babies.

Soreness Abounds: Pull Your Nipples Into the Car When Driving

Before working on latching or comfort positioning, it's important to avoid having nipples that look like they've been dragged up a busy street, hanging out the car door. If your nipples are already cracked, sore, and extremely irritated, breastfeeding, if not done deeply, may add insult to injury, and your nipples will continue to hurt. If I'm too late in pointing this out, you need some of Dr. Jack Newman's APNO (All Purpose Nipple Ointment). Obtaining this prescription should be fairly easy if you're able to tell your practitioner both the ingredients and the amounts that comprise APNO. It would be unfair (and unwise) of you to expect your practitioner to go research this in the middle of your baby's newborn visit. According to Dr. Newman's website (Newman, 2010), the recipe contains:

- The antibiotic: bactroban (mupirocin) 2% ointment (not cream): 15 grams.

- The anti-inflammatory: betamethasone 0.1% ointment (not cream): 15 grams.

- The anti-fungal: miconazole powder, so the final concentration is 2% miconazole.

You can also try a pair of hydrogel dressings (like Soothies), and you'll feel like your nipples just had an epidural. I'm especially fond of hydrogel dressings because they support moist wound healing by forming a protective barrier over the wound. This allows the tissue to heal without scabbing. If scabs form, the baby usually sucks them off at the next feeding, and then the entire healing process has to start again.

Please don't confuse this with keeping the breast WET, which can lead to a breast that looks like it has severe diaper rash...

Baby's Weight Loss: What's Important and What's Normal

Babies can and usually do lose from 7-10% of their birth weights. We call the lowest weight your baby drops to his "nadir weight." This is normal. Weight gain AFTER birth should always be measured from this nadir or lowest weight, which usually occurs on the third or fourth day. Make sure you write down or remember baby's discharge weight from the hospital and compare it to your baby's weight at the first visit in the pediatrician's office.

Calculating weight loss is easy. If your baby weighed 7 pounds, 1 ounce at birth, multiply 7 pounds times 16 ounces (since there are 16 ounces in a pound) to get 112, then add the one ounce to get 113 ounces. To easily calculate 10 percent of that, move the decimal point one digit to the left of the whole number, to 11.3 ounces. Then subtract the 10 percent from baby's birthweight. This would equal 6 lbs, 6 oz. This number is the lowest acceptable weight loss you should have in a newborn.

If baby's weight is more than that number (in this case, more than 6 lbs, 6 oz), great! If it's less than 6 lbs, 6 oz, you probably need to do some extra feedings to catch-up. If your baby now weighs 6 lbs, 6 oz or less, this is the weight loss where we usually start supplementing a small amount of breastmilk, donor milk, or formula (about an ounce) at either every feeding or every other feeding. Having said this, there are a lot of factors involved with this decision, and one we will partially explore later on in the book.

It's not a coincidence that mom's milk increases at the same time baby reaches the nadir weight, so if mom's milk has just "come in" or become more plentiful, then I delay supplementing, providing the baby looks good and healthy. I ask mom to feed like crazy and return to the office the next day for a weight check.

Really, the first 40 days postpartum is a time when a mom's body is primed and ready to make milk. This is when emptying the breast and having effective breast drainage is paramount to milk production (Mohrbacher, 2010). I call this maximizing your potential for milk production.

If the weight loss is between 7-10% and baby is jaundiced (making them too sleepy to suck at times), a good hospital-grade electric pump might be helpful.

Because breasts aren't that smart, we need to help them continue to produce milk. Pumping both breasts at one time, immediately after a breastfeeding (or while formula feeding if your supply isn't established), will make the breasts think you had twins. Your breastfeeding hormones (prolactin and oxytocin) will increase, and the breasts will snap to attention. It may take about five days to really start to see some decent results, so don't panic. I'm partial to a hospital-grade pump; don't try to get away with using one that's store-bought. The pump does make a difference if baby is not spending much time at the breast.

Babies become more and more efficient eaters as time goes by, and, therefore, breastfeeding becomes easier for moms. Lactation experts note that, by the end of the first week, a mother's milk production has increased more than 10-fold—from an average of a little more than one ounce (37-56 ml) per day total on the first day to a little over 20 ounces by day seven (Neville et al., 1988), with women who breastfed a previous baby being one day ahead (Ingram, Woolridge, Greenwood, & McGrath, 1999). By the second and third weeks, babies can hold about two to three ounces per feed and take about 20-25 ounces of milk per day (Mohrbacher, 2010).

Appropriate Infant Weight Gain: Introducing the "No Schedule" Schedule

After baby hits his nadir weight (rock bottom weight on day three or four), he should start gaining about an ounce a day. This is an important number. Weight should be checked within a few days after the first pediatrician's office appointment to make sure it's all on the upswing. As a number to keep in your mind, we're looking for roughly two pounds a month for the first few months.

In my clinical practice, despite my urgings for moms to have confidence and follow their instincts, I'll occasionally have a woman for whom this just doesn't seem to be working. I've even had a mother look me squarely in the face and scream, "Dammit Kathy, just tell me what to do!"

With that in mind, this is the part of the book I write for moms who have honestly tried to rely on their instincts and still have not made the progress they'd like to be making. I think of it like a jump-start when your car battery is low.

Here are some thoughts if you think your baby is hungry and you're not producing enough milk. Pump both breasts (hospital-grade pump) at once for 20-30 minutes. You can either do this after a feeding (short or long, one side or both), instead of a feeding, or WHILE you're feeding (meaning baby on one breast and pump on the other). Yes, I know what kind of time commitment this is, but remember, this is short term, and we already had that warrior talk.

This is a NO SCHEDULE schedule. This means YOU decide the best time and way to accomplish this. Keep a baby's natural rhythm in mind by remembering how often they feed and how they also cluster feed.

To increase supply, you can even consider keeping the pump in a place where you pass by frequently, and do a quick 5-10 minute pumping each time you pass. No need to clean the pieces after each pumping, as breastmilk is good left out for six hours. Leave the milk there and just keep adding to it (Mohrbacher, 2010).

To increase supply, you can also go to bed with your baby for 24 hours.....lots of skin-to-skin and snuggling can work wonders.

The Draconian (Meaning Harsh, Rigorous, or Severe) Schedule

Schedules are really a thing of the past. We previously gave mothers very intense schedules and directions to follow. What we discovered is that babies did just as well when we allowed moms to decide when their infants needed to eat...... Who would have thought??? Having said this, in my clinical practice, I still have moms asking me for more direction until they can tap into their own thoughts and methods. I still have babies who have lost 7-10% or more of their birthweight and have difficulty gaining the one ounce a day. For those exhausted, frustrated mothers and those situations, this is what I tell them they can TRY. It's also the exact schedule I gave to the mom who clearly stated to "just tell me what to do." This draconian schedule is a two-day trial to jump-start your breasts in cases where baby is not up to the task.

- 7:00 a.m. (or whenever your day starts) - Breastfeed using one breast for 5-10 minutes. Supplement the baby with ½-1 ounce of formula (only if there is no real production of breastmilk when pumping). Pump both breasts for 20 minutes, and save this milk to use at the next session to top-off baby after either the next nursing or feeding cue.

- 9:00 a.m. - Breastfeed using the other breast for 5-10 minutes. (If the baby is doing beautifully and gulping with gusto, go ahead and nurse as long as you want, and use both breasts). Listen for audible swallows, and be aware if the other breast is leaking. Supplement the baby with the milk you expressed at 7:00 a.m. You may need to use a bit of formula if you were not able to express enough milk. Let others do the bottle-feeding when possible. You can't do it all! Finish by pumping both breasts for 20 minutes.

- Repeat the 9:00 a.m. process every 2-2½ hours throughout the day. Pick two times, perhaps 11:00 a.m. and 5:00 p.m., when all you do is pump for 20-30 minutes. This way, Dad or Grandma will have some expressed milk and can help you with feedings.

- At night (after your bedtime, around 10:00-11:00 p.m.), try to get one three-hour break and one four-hour break. It doesn't matter whether the longer break or shorter break comes first. If it all starts to fall apart at night and you're feeling exhausted and disheartened, feed the baby a couple ounces of formula (while you pump once in the middle of the night) and get back to sleep.

As your milk comes in and your baby is audibly swallowing, as well as pooping yellow, seedy stools (like mustard with pesto bits in it, as one father described it), pull back on pumping and just breastfeed. When your baby is back to his birthweight, you can stop waking him at night. Continue with the frequent feedings during the day, as the baby needs to have 8-10 feedings per day.

Infants who are allowed to sleep all day will be awake all night. Count on it! They're resting up for the party and you're invited. If left to their own devices, they'll become nocturnal. That's why, if baby is repeatedly up all night long, feeding fewer times than eight times in 24 hours or not gaining as much as they should, it's important to wake them during the day. In other words, don't let them have that one long four- to five-hour stretch during the day.

In all my years of practice, I only had one mom (a nurse that worked nights), who loved the fact that her baby slept while she did during the day. This way, the poor babysitter was the one dealing with an awake baby all night. They spent from 3:00-11:00 p.m. in the evenings bonding and having the best part of their days. I often wonder what happened as that little guy grew up? Perhaps they had to move to another time zone at some point.

It's not my favorite thing to recommend moms use formula and breastpumps, but sometimes, in order to preserve the breastfeeding relationship, moms need a little break and help while they're establishing a milk supply. Follow your heart here, as there is no clear right and wrong answer—only what works for you and your baby.

If you can bring your milk in and baby back to birth weight by two weeks of age, gaining about an ounce a day with exclusive breastfeeding, that's ALWAYS preferable. I have, however, worked with many parents who need some alternative thoughts on how to get the job done. It is for this reason that I include these other methods.

Signs of Dryness: Brick Dust in the Diaper - Attention K-Mart Shoppers!

Newborn babies can get mildly dehydrated pretty quickly because they don't have the reserve you and I do. When you see a pinkish orange smear (like brick dust) in the diaper, what in medical-speak we call "urate crystals," it means your baby is getting pretty thirsty/hungry. You should try frequent breastfeedings and/or pumping to give the baby more milk for less work or supplement a bit more with formula (if you're formula feeding). You might also notice the baby's lips are chapped or there isn't much moisture in the mouth. To help the chapping as you're feeding more, you can put some breastmilk or a tiny amount of Vaseline right on the baby's lips. Advise your healthcare provider about the brick dust. This is not necessarily an emergency, so no middle of the night calls. You just need to increase baby's intake.

Basket of Rolls to Delay the Shark's Feeding Frenzy

Think about what it's like being very hungry and sitting down at a restaurant. What's the first thing you do? "Waiter! Can we please have some rolls?" Sometimes you just can't wait for the entrée and need a little nibble in order to relax and eat like a lady. Babies sometimes can't settle into their latch because they're frantically hungry, which can look like he can't decide whether he wants to eat or not. You may have to offer baby a half-ounce bottle of expressed breastmilk or formula (preferably breastmilk), just so he can get a grip.

What if, after all this nonsense with the basket of rolls, the baby still won't restart eating? If he takes a few sucks, and then comes off the breast, that's okay, too. Maybe he's actually finished and just wanted a dessert suck. You can use this time to pump (if you have any reason to do so) or to take a break and burp the baby. You can also change the diaper or clean the belly button. Then offer your baby the other side. With babies, there's always something to do. Just don't try to hurry a feeding or delay a feeding too often, as babies can feel the stress and anxiety coming from you.

I'm frequently asked if Mom can give her baby the basket of rolls/supplemental bottle, or if it should ideally be someone else. My answer is that it should ideally be someone else. When baby thinks Mom, he should think breast. He shouldn't have to ask, "What do you want me to suck on today, mom? Breast, bottle, finger?" I say ideally, because if you're home alone, then you have to be the one to do it. We can also have baby finish on the breast after the basket of rolls, which will have babies associate the breast with a full tummy.

Am I Feeding My Baby Enough or Is He Just Going for the Dessert Cart?

Don't assume that babies need to eat as much breastmilk as formula. Studies show that four-month-old babies who eat formula, eat, on average, 33% more milk per day than breastfed babies (Neville et al., 1991). Therefore, moms can rest assured that they do NOT need to pump as much milk as a baby will eat when baby drinks formula. The reasons for this are varied and have to do with how babies take the breasts (slowly), as well as the differences in the milk itself (Mohrbacher, 2010).

So, babies will usually take more milk by bottle, whether breastmilk or formula, because it's non-stop flow. Babies are overly full by the time they know to stop eating because of how quickly the milk comes out. We know this because, when breastfeeding, babies take less volume and always leave some milk in their mom's breasts, so we know it's not an availability problem.

Here's the most important piece of feeding information you need to know: If babies are gaining weight adequately, you don't need to make more milk. Babies can thrive beautifully on different amounts of milk AND babies needs do NOT usually increase the amount you supply after the first five weeks. There's more to weight gain than how much milk babies take.

When moms tell me that their babies are always willing to take more food after they nurse, they mistakenly think that means they NEED that food. I explain this by asking if mom ever eats more than she's hungry for, just because the dessert cart comes around at the end of a wonderful restaurant meal. So, the idea being that sometimes babies eat more than what they're hungry for, too.

It's very important to note that, despite rapid growth spurts, the amount of milk a breastfed baby takes a day, between one and six months of age, remains remarkably stable (Mohrbacher, 2010).

Burping (at the Bar)

There are lots of ways to burp your baby... ask anyone. My personal favorite is called "Burping at the Bar." I like it for two reasons: you can see your baby's face and mouth, and you don't get spit-up down your back. Parents often think they need to spend a lot more time here than is necessary. It's OK to give it a minute or two, and then move on. Think about burping whenever baby gets fidgety at the breast or keeps coming off the breast.

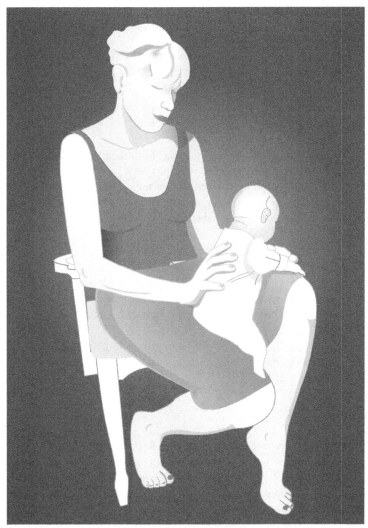

Figure 1.11 Burping at the Bar

For this position, you need to sit down and raise your left knee by bringing your left foot up on your toes. That's the bar. Now with your lower right knee about two inches away, sit the baby on the lower knee. This is the barstool. Remember that when you burp, you should concentrate on the baby's left side because that's where the stomach is located. Make an alligator hand (like you're mimicking a mouth) to grab the left side of the baby and gently squeeze up.

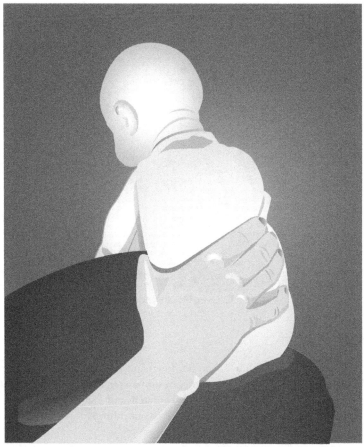

Figure 1.12 Alligator Hand

You should get a burp very quickly. If not, try some gentle rubbing. I'm not a fan of gently pounding the baby to get a burp. It seems to only contribute to reflux. Other burping positions that generally work well are using the colic hold (no patting or rubbing required (illustrated in Chapter 8, figure 8.1) and the classic, over-the-shoulder hold (with some specific twists).

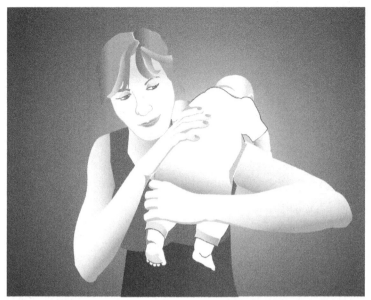

Figure 1.13 Over-the-Shoulder Burping

Out in Public?

When it's time to eat, it's time to eat. Sit down and feed your baby wherever you are. Many states now have laws that protect a woman's right to breastfeed in public. Online, you can check out the National Conference of State Legislatures (2010) for a state-by-state listing of laws and miscellaneous information on breastfeeding.

Most women are able to breastfeed discreetly, but there are some people in the community that, believe it or not, are still offended. In a society where there's a lot of pressure to be politically correct, I find it amazing how strangers are still quite comfortable in offering their decidedly non-politically correct thoughts. It would be nice to socialize these people, so be fearless and confident in the fact that you are doing the best thing for your baby. Remember that breastfeeding is completely normal and natural, and the more women breastfeed in public, the more people will realize this.

For the first time mom, breastfeeding in public may not come naturally. You've had a lifetime of keeping your breasts hidden, and it can take time to get used to using them in public. With preparation, practice, and breastfeeding support, though, you can boost your confidence. If you are self-conscious and want to make sure you are concealing your breast and feeding to your baby's and your comfort level, you can practice at home with a blanket, breastfeeding cover, carrier, or sling. When you get to the place where you know you are going to nurse, it might be helpful to really evaluate where you are—you can request a seat out of the way in a restaurant or look for designated breastfeeding places while out shopping. You can also seek out support in the form of consultations with experts – your nurse practitioner, doctor, midwife, and/or lactation consultant, and in groups with other breastfeeding mothers – at hospital or private breastfeeding centers and your local La Leche League meetings. Lastly, be aware that when people stare or jeer at you, it is really saying more about that person than about you or what you're doing. People may be giving you looks because they are inappropriately sexualizing your life-sustaining breast, or they may be uncomfortable with their own body or feeding choices.

Breasts have many meanings for people. During an office visit with me, one dad was becoming very uncomfortable with me touching his wife's breasts. He finally said, "If I knew you were going to touch my wife like that, I would have left the room." He also didn't want to be in the waiting room if a woman was breastfeeding, and would ask to be taken back to a private exam room where he wouldn't be exposed to such "indecencies."

Of course, the universe has a way of taking care of people like this. The couple worked for the State Department, and their next post was in Africa. The father went first for a few months to scout new housing, and took a village bus into the next town, a three-hour trip. On the way, the woman sitting next to him had a two-year-old on her lap who got a bit hungry. She took her breast out and proceeded to feed for the entire trip. By the time they reached their destination, he was totally desensitized. He was so proud as he told me this story a couple of years later when they came back to Washington to have their next baby—he seemed like an entirely different dad!

I also had an Australian mom in my practice with an interesting story about breastfeeding in public. She had just moved to the U.S. after her fifth child was born. She was amazed at all the differences in just about every aspect of living here. One day, she went shopping at a "gourmet grocery store" that specialized in whole and organic foods. While shopping she literally was lost in time (because she was staring at both the beauty of the food and the prices) and started getting engorged. She promptly went to the customer service counter and asked if they had a chair where she could feed her baby.

The store manager came rushing to her aid, bringing his own office chair (the kind with wheels) to the front of the store and put her right in the front window, a beautiful sunny spot. She promptly started taking her breast out of her blouse. He came charging back, asking her what she was doing, all the while starting to wheel her to the bathroom behind a fruit display. He didn't even let her get out of the chair. She was flabbergasted. He said, "You can't do that here, lady. This isn't that kind of a store!" I guess they didn't mean that kind of natural and organic store. As she recanted this story to me, her comment was that "Americans sure are a strange group of people." Sometimes, I agree.

Chapter 2

Your Breasts (at Least They Used to Be) and Your Milk (the Holy Grail)

Porn Star or Primary Engorgement?

Hopefully, around day three to six, you'll wake up knowing your milk is in. This is called "Primary Engorgement." Your breasts will feel full. It can be a bit difficult to get the baby to latch onto your bigger, harder breasts. By frequent breastfeeding, you can avoid having the breasts get to the point (pun intended) where they're unrecognizable. Imagine trying to bite into a stale loaf of bread. An important first step is to soften the areola, then you can sandwich the breast, so the baby can easily start to suckle. Sub sandwiches are often too big to fit into your mouth. They need to be compressed, so you can take a bite. You can compress the areola a bit by getting just a little milk out before you start to feed the baby. You can do this by hand expression, reverse pressure softening (described below), or with a breastpump (manual or electric).

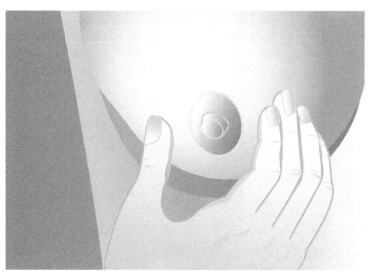

2.1. Hand Expression

If simply expressing some milk isn't helping the latch during engorgement, there are many other methods to try. These include breastfeeding with the baby tummy down on your body while you're semi-reclined, wearing breast shells about a half hour before feeding to help soften the areola (you can buy these at a baby store or from your lactation consultant), and short-term use of a nipple shield to help the baby latch onto something. Breast massage after applying heat for a minute or two may help soften the breasts as well.

Ow, Ow, OOOWWW! Yes, in addition to experiencing difficulty latching, engorgement can be painful to YOU as well. You can use any and all of the following to combat the pain:

- Take NSAIDS (e.g., Ibuprofen or Naproxen) or Tylenol.

- Use cold compresses.

- Breastfeed often and long.

- Express your milk by hand expression or pump just until you are comfortable if your breasts are still full after breastfeeding.

Another important strategy in softening the areola is called "Reverse Pressure Softening." This method involves using gentle, but consistent pressure around the nipple. The RPS method (Cotterman, 2004) was developed by nurse Jean Cotterman to be used ANYTIME an areola needs softening. One website explaining the procedure in detail with diagrams is www.kellymom.com. This is a method that can easily be googled.

Occasionally, moms will feel a golf ball-sized lump in their armpits. This tissue extending into the armpit is called the Tail of Spence and is simply engorged breast tissue. Yup, your milk comes in all the way up there. Nothing special you need to do except wait it out and use cold compresses if it makes you feel more comfortable.

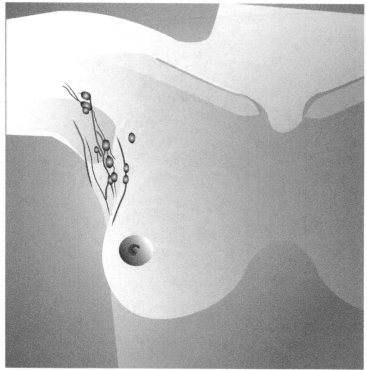
Figure 2.2 Tail of Spence

Cabbage Trick: Not Just for the Polish

If you can't get the bowling balls calmed down and they're still hurting, go to the store (read: send somebody to the store) and buy a nice head of green cabbage. Break off the leaves whole (two at a time), rinse them in cold water, blot dry, strip the large vein and roll over them with a rolling pin between two pieces of wax paper. Place one in each side of your bra (yes, you heard me correctly) and save the rest in the refrigerator. Also remember to leave the nipples exposed by cutting a whole in the center of the leaf. When they wilt after a few hours, replace them. You should see results within about three changes. A scientific explanation as to why cabbage leaves are effective would be nice, but, unfortunately, there is none. You'll just have to trust me on this one, it works.

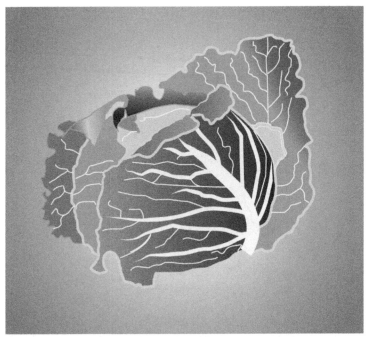

Figure 2.3 Cabbage

Thanks for the Mammaries... or Hot Dog Rolls or Big Girl Bras? You Decide

You will feel much more comfortable during your postpartum days if your breasts are up and supported by a well-fitting, "big-girl" bra. Frankly, you'll look better (neater, thinner, and more comfortable) in clothes as well. Your breasts might change sizes a couple of times as your milk becomes more plentiful, so you might have to go through the process of finding a well-fitting bra more than once. If possible, try to get professionally fitted at a high-end bra shop. I know, it is another indignity you need to endure, but it has to be less exposing than showing your goods during labor, and you survived that just fine. Your bra fitter is typically an older lady that has seen more breasts than a lantern on Bourbon Street in New Orleans. Hopefully, she won't yell to the other salesperson across the crowded showroom floor from your dressing room, *"BLANCHE, you got any more of those Triple Z's in the back? This lady just leaked all over this one."* This reminds me, bring nursing pads to your fitting session.

You can, of course, try to find a well-fitting bra on your own. If your breasts are poking out, there is side-spillage, or the underwire cuts into your breast tissue anywhere, you need to go up a cup size. A well-fitting bra fits well on the loosest hook, and it should not cut into your skin. If your breasts are particularly pendulous, you might need wider straps for more support. Make sure you try a shirt on over your bra with breast pads, if you wear them, to assess whether the appearance is smooth enough.

You don't necessarily need to purchase expensive nursing shirts, but your breasts should be accessible to your baby by wearing front-opening button-ups or something you can easily pull down or to the side. It never ceases to amaze me when breastfeeding mothers come to our pediatric office wearing a dress. Dresses look great because they hide the postpartum tummy. But in order to breastfeed, they have to be taken off completely. It's also helpful to wear a sleep bra (one without metal hooks or plastic clips) or a camisole (with a built-in bra) to bed or anytime you'd like to lie down and sleep. The bra/camisole will keep the breasts together without flapping around the bed, which would cause them to feel uncomfortable and make more milk.

Your breasts have gone through a lot of changes, and will go through more, as you continue to breastfeed. Although it is logical that you or your partner may currently view your breasts as more utilitarian than anything else, appearance and feeling "sexy" are still key to feeling good about yourself. When I finished breastfeeding two kids, I didn't know whether to buy bras or hot dog rolls. Breasts can start to look like tube socks with a golf ball in the toe. The degree of sagginess or misshapenness is not so much related to breastfeeding itself, but rather more to genetics, hormones secreted during pregnancy, and, yes, the wearing of well-fitting, supportive bras while lactating.

My final thought on postpartum bodies is that you may want to consider wearing something with light support around your tummy. SPANX works, as do postpartum supports (like a girdle, but with mild support), you just need something to help re-teach the broad ligaments supporting you internally. I'm not talking about looking like a movie star, just about taking care of your body and avoiding an uncomfortable feeling.

Big Boobs – Grand Tetons: She's Got a Balcony You Can Do Shakespeare From!

Yes, you know who you are…the woman who is making her way through the alphabet in bra sizes. You were big boobed before pregnancy, and now, with nursing, you are just humongously top heavy. You have to shop in specialty stores or lactation centers to find a bra in your size, and you face different challenges than your nursing friends who are less endowed. Your breasts might or might not seem like Jugs of Joy to you, but they are beautiful in what they provide for your baby. And no, you won't smother your baby with your large breasts, but big breasts do require special upkeep or else some complications might arise.

Many friends will tell you that it is so easy to nurse lying down in bed, and you and your child will sleep better for it. For you well-endowed girls, the traditional lie down on your side with your back propped position may not work. I found that for some larger breasted women, using the breast that is actually not closest to the bed, propped up on a cushion, may be more comfortable for feeding while lying down than using the breast on the bottom.

As a large breasted breastfeeding woman, you need to keep your breasts supported adequately, or you can experience pain in your breasts. I had one big–breasted (cup size H) patient for whom a doctor and I initially treated for thrush, when in actuality, it turned out that she was suffering from torn ligaments in her breasts. Her excruciating, unexplainable, both-sided pain while breastfeeding really indicated to me that she had thrush. Her pain symptoms were exacerbated by the fact that she had been instructed to "air out" her breasts (i.e., go braless) as much as possible as part of the protocol for thrush. In this case, though, the hours the patient was not wearing a bra further contributed to stretched and torn ligaments in her breast. Once she wore a well-supported bra 24 hours a day for a week, the pain started to subside. For big-breasted women, it is important to wear a well-fitting bra 24-7, and to endure a professional bra fitting to ensure a proper fit. Those "sleep bras" for breastfeeding really do not provide enough adequate support for large breasts, even overnight.

When pumping, do keep in mind that flange sizes correspond to NIPPLE sizes and not breast size, so you could possibly fit into a small flange, even though you have large breasts.

When you are breastfeeding with big breasts, it is also important to make sure you bring your baby up to where your breast should be or is when the breast is supported in a bra, and not push your breast down or let your breast hang down to your baby. You might have to be on the lookout for chairs with armrests to support your elbow, while you raise and support your breast with your hand to feed your baby.

Your Milk

It's so common to have women place blame on themselves for everything that could be going wrong (even when it's not). Moms tell me they don't have enough milk to feed their baby, or their milk isn't rich enough or thick enough. If men breastfed, they'd be erecting monuments to their bosoms and copious milk supplies. Relax.

Breast size has nothing to do with how much milk moms can make. Production and storage capacity are determined by the amount of glandular tissue moms have. Until you start breastfeeding, you just don't know how much milk you'll be able to make and store. This is just one piece to look at in determining how often your baby will feed and whether you'll always need both breasts or just one at every feeding (Mohrbacher, 2010).

One question I've been asked over and over again is, "Why does one breast make more milk than the other?" "Should I try to even things up?" My answer is always the same. One breast might have more glandular tissue or more milk pores, but whatever the reason, it's not important and you don't need to do anything about it. It's the overall supply babies care about, not which breast makes more.

Boy That's Nothing or What a *Letdown*!

Breasts are never empty. You can have several letdown reflexes or "MERs" (Milk-Ejection Reflexes) during the course of a feeding or pumping. You may feel none, you may feel only the first, or you may feel all of them. Each letdown will involve both breasts and last an average of two minutes (Prime, Geddes, & Hartmann, 2007). Describing the feeling of the letdown is like describing an orgasm, meaning it's going to be different for everybody. Some mothers describe it as feeling like pins and needles, almost like the breast is falling asleep. Others describe it as feeling like their breast is being squeezed in a vice. It's all normal.

Letdown is exactly what it sounds like--your milk letting down from your breasts into your baby's mouth. It usually occurs about a minute into feeding, and you should hear baby swallowing audibly when this happens. If pumping, you'll definitely see the milk squirting into the flanges. Letdown usually occurs three to four times during a breastfeeding, with a range of 1 to 17 (Cobo, 1993; Kent et al., 2008). Pumping yields approximately the same number of letdowns as a breastfeeding (Ramsay, Kent, Owens & Hartmann, 2004).

If you are curious about exactly where the milk comes out, there are between 4 and 18 nipple openings (or pores) (Ramsay, Kent, Owens, & Hartmann, 2005) on the end of each nipple, and six to eight alternate openings when your milk lets down. It's like a little showerhead!

You may want to have a big glass of water handy when breastfeeding. My niece, an Iowa farm girl, said that the second her milk would let down she wanted to stick her head in a trough and drink it all up—now that's a thirsty letdown!

Breastfeeding Diet: Not!

The good news here is that there is no breastfeeding diet you have to stick to, no real restrictions that you need. This isn't an illness! Yes, you can have coffee, all fruits and vegetables, and alcohol (in moderation and NOT every night). Just remember that whatever you put in your mouth, you put in baby's mouth. This means YOU have to pay attention to what agrees with you and your baby and what doesn't.

If you visit an Indian restaurant and order extra spicy food that gives YOU gas, don't be surprised if the baby has gas, too. A simethicone product (like Mylicon Infant Drops, Phazyme, or Little Tummies) can be used as directed to help baby pass gas painlessly. A word of caution is that some parents and practitioners think these products do absolutely nothing. Ultimately, YOU should be the judge of that. Many people believe products sold for baby's gas will simply stop it, but it is just meant to relieve the surface tension on the gas bubbles, POSSIBLY alleviating some of the pain. There are moms that swear by it.

Babies tell you they have painful gas by pulling their legs up, screaming, and passing gas. You'll wish you had stayed home from the restaurant and dined on boiled chicken and rice. You'll need to experiment. If you run across a food that agrees with you, but doesn't agree with baby, wait a month and try it again. You'll also want to do your experimenting as early in the day as possible, so the baby can still sleep comfortably that night.

Food you have eaten can take anywhere from about 30 minutes to 24 hours to reach your breastmilk. Alcohol peaks in milk in 30 to 90 minutes. Medications are usually faster at seeping into your breastmilk, depending on the type of medication (i.e., the dosage, how quickly it goes to work, how it's metabolized, etc.). The baby's pediatric practice should be made aware of ANY medication mom is taking while breastfeeding. Many offices have resources, like Thomas Hale's (2010) *Medications and Mothers' Milk*, which will inform parents on safety issues.

In my clinical practice, the number one food that seems to cause the most problems in infants is DAIRY....I'm talking dairy in every form: milk, cheese, yogurt, ice cream, pudding and butter.

I know it is difficult to take dairy foods out of your diet because they're girl foods. If you think dairy foods might be the culprit, try eliminating these foods for one week to see if it makes a difference.

Exercise, Wait a Bit, and Use the German Bra: Holdsem'fromfloppin

I can't say enough positive things about how much exercise helps your mood and your body.

It also relieves stress, and who doesn't need that?

It's a known fact that when we exercise to exhaustion, our muscles produce lactic acid. Simply put, lactic acid, when mixed with breastmilk, can taste bad. Babies MAY refuse to nurse after your vigorous workout. You may need to pump immediately before you start, wear a supportive sports bra, and then wait for an hour after exercising for the lactic acid to be reabsorbed. Having said that, you can also just exercise and breastfeed, and see how it works for you, as every mother/

baby couple is unique. The latest clinical research we have on this shows that the lactic acid concentrations after exercising is not likely to be a problem for most moms (Dewey & McCrory, 1994; Wright, Quinn, & Carey, 2002).

Breastpads

Although cloth pads are more cost effective, they can get pretty cold and uncomfortable when wet, so you'll have to change them frequently. If you buy disposable pads, get the ones with the sticky adhesive strip on the back, so you're not reaching into your shirt to reposition one that just slipped north or south of the border.

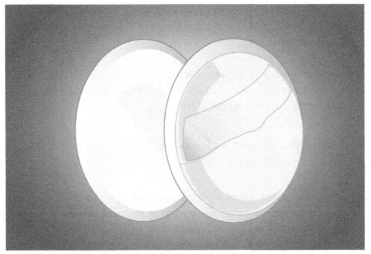

Figure 2.4 Breastpads

Oversupply: Hey, Turn That Hose Off!

Some moms may have too much breastmilk. When you have an oversupply, your breasts are always heavy and full, and your milk lets down with a vengeance. Your baby may sputter and choke after the first few minutes of breastfeeding, trying to keep up with the "fire hose" in his mouth. Babies cope with this by arching their backs and pulling back, biting, or chomping down to help slow the flow of milk. They'll have incredible weight gain, can be fussy between nursings, and appear to be perpetually hungry. My personal thoughts on this is because they get so gassy, they try to comfort themselves by sucking, only to get more milk. It's also been proposed that because the baby cannot ever reach the hindmilk (fattier milk), they never feel satisfied. These babies also usually have noisy, explosive poops. If this sounds familiar, don't despair. There are several solutions.

Keep in mind that your milk production is usually on a "supply and demand" schedule. If you just use one breast per feeding, this will cause the other breast to calm down since it's only being used every four hours or so. There is a type of feeding called "Block Feeding." Moms double pump early in the day to empty the breasts, and then use one breast per block of time (like four to six hours). You must be vigilant in watching your milk supply if you try any of these methods. If you plan on using this method, consult a lactation consultant for more information and various methods.

As an alternative, you can feed with baby in a more dominant position to the breast. Placing baby on top of you, while lying back, can make feeding much more comfortable for both of you. You might get a bit of a milk bath, so be prepared with a small burp cloth. When baby is not clamping down as much, your nipples should start to feel much better. Nipple shields, which look like a silicone sombrero for a mouse, can be helpful to work as a governor when you do breastfeed in the mommy-dominant position.

You can also try sucking on peppermint Altoids or taking ONE Sudafed, which may be more than enough. As a last resort, try the cabbage trick for a few hours one day, and repeat for a second day if necessary.

Undersupply...Where's the beef????? Errrrrr...I Mean Milk

Too little milk can be worse than too much milk because you're left with a hungry baby, alternating between crying and staring at your breasts. Since breastmilk is based on supply and demand, there shouldn't be a problem, but there can be. The reasons are incredibly varied and range from losing too much blood (right after the delivery with postpartum hemorrhage), to simply not putting your baby to the breast often enough. Since it takes three to five days to establish a milk supply, well-meaning nursery personnel might have quieted the baby in the nursery with a nice, big bottle of formula. A big downfall of this practice is how it raises expectations for infants in terms of how much food is to be delivered at one time. Since your breasts didn't need to make as much milk the day or days your baby was supplemented, your supply might have started off lower.

Other factors contributing to low milk production are:

- No breast changes during pregnancy or experiencing no breast fullness and/or engorgement after birth
- Hypoplastic breast
- Retained placenta (where moms continue to bleed longer than normal)
- Birth control pills
- Thyroid issues

- Polycystic Ovarian Syndrome (PCOS)

These issues need to be addressed with your clinician. There are also cases that have no obvious cause.

If no underlying medical issue is found or treated, you need a "galactogogue," a big word that refers to a product that will help increase your milk production. Put the word into the Google search engine and start reading. In the meantime, here's a quick list of products that will/may "help:"

- *Reglan – Metoclopramide.* (A prescription drug that was once prescribed to help with acid reflux also has this strange side effect of increasing mom's milk....10mg, three times a day for seven days).

- *Domperidone - Motillum.* Another reflux product. This can be obtained over the Internet from countries outside the U.S. or from a compounding pharmacy in the U.S. The usual dose ranges from 10 to 20 mg three times daily. Do not use this if you have cardiac problems, particularly arrhythmias. Do your homework prior to taking this product and discuss it with your practitioner. There is an FDA warning.

- *Fenugreek.* - This is sold under names like Mothers Milk Tea. Some women swear by it; others curse the taste and hold their noses. My personal feeling is that it couldn't hurt, and many mothers have claimed overwhelming success.

- *Oatmeal.* Self-explanatory...the product that is, not why it works. Use steel-cut oats, like McCann's, and prepare according to directions on the box. A nice, warm bowl in the morning has been reported to increase supply on the day it's eaten. Some possible explanations are that it increases iron levels, decreases cholesterol, and is comforting to moms (comfort=relaxation=better milk flow). At any rate, although never scientifically proven, it just might work for you. Anyway, the worst that can happen is you'll have a nutritious breakfast.

Using any of the above products does not get you off the hook from doing your homework with breastfeeding basics. You should still check the baby's latch and increase pumping and/or feeding. Galactogogues are not meant to be a silver bullet cure, but rather something you can try in addition to other things.

The Breastfeeding Mother's Guide to Making More Milk is an excellent resource for dosages and quality sources of herbal remedies for increasing milk. U.S. lactation consultants Diana West and Lisa Marasco (2009), authors of the book, have also created a website - www.lowmilksupply.org/herbalgalactagogues.shtml.

Two other wonderful resources for many aspects of breastfeeding, in addition to low milk supply, are www.mobimotherhood.org and www.mother-food.com. The latter describes itself as a "wonderful collection of historical traditions from cultures around the world and what they feed mothers to support good health, breastfeeding, and plentiful milk production."

Human Milk Fortifier, from the makers of Enfamil formula, is like Hamburger Helper for breastmilk. It's a product you can give to your baby mixed with your milk. This powder comes in small serving size packets that you sprinkle into expressed breastmilk. It increases the caloric content (two to four calories per ounce depending on how you mix it) to help the baby gain weight. You can ask your friendly pharmacist to order it over the counter. No prescription is required. With this product, you can make the milk you do have be more efficient.

Supplemental Nursing System and the Lactaid

The point of the "at breast supplementers" is to have your baby get his nutritional needs met with formula, donor milk, or your previously expressed milk, while you bond with your baby by breastfeeding. It also allows your breasts to be stimulated, increasing your supply. This is a good solution for adoptive moms who want the benefits of having baby at the breast. The supplementer looks like a flask (filled with milk) that you hang between your breasts. The flask has two tubes coming from the bottom, which curve back over your breasts onto your nipples. When the baby suckles the breast, he also gets a piece of tubing in his mouth that feeds some formula. Voila!

Before purchasing one, do your homework to decide which at breast supplementer is best for you and your baby. They both have pluses and minuses.

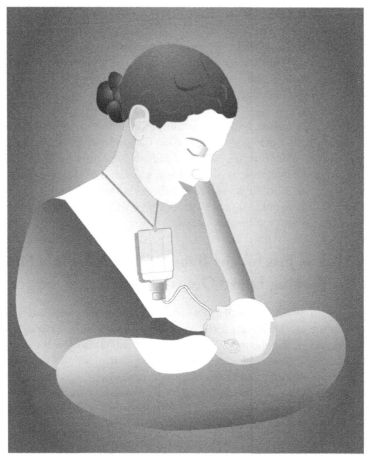

Figure 2.5 SNS

Both Breast and Bottle

Moms sometimes choose breastfeeding and formula, thinking they're giving the baby their precious milk, while giving themselves a break. Although this is not my favorite choice because any amount of formula feeding affects your breastmilk supply, I can instruct you on how to do it. Any amount of breastfeeding is always better than no breastfeeding. I always like mothers to be well informed when they make a decision. You can decide to do whatever you want, but do it from a position of knowledge.

According to the "prolactin receptor theory" (de Carvalho, Robertson, Friedman, & Klaus, 1983), there are a critical two weeks after birth to establish a good milk supply. During this time, mothers increase milk supply potential by raising their prolactin levels and, therefore, activating more receptors in their breasts to make milk. How do you raise your prolactin level? Simple. Drain your breasts well and often by either breastfeeding or pumping.

This means that if you decide you want to also use formula, it's better to start after your own milk supply is fully established. At that point if you want to try formula, start with about an ounce in the early morning (make sure you pump your breasts if you're within the first fourteen days) to see how well it agrees with your baby. Some babies will vomit, some will sleep awhile longer, some will sleep less, some may develop a rash, and others will show no changes.

When babies are given both breastmilk and formula, it affects the stool and digestive tract. Formula washes away good bacteria from the inside of the intestines. It takes two full weeks to re-cultivate the bacteria. Inside the intestines, you'll find quickly moving breastmilk followed by slower moving formula. Formula makes some babies gassy, while other babies do quite well. Additionally, formula stays in the gut longer than breastmilk, so it will wreak havoc with your schedule when the baby's not hungry and your breasts are full.

This Milk Is Just for the Baby—Older Children Should Not Be Washing Down Oreos With It

This may be an obvious point, but I once had a home visit where the baby was not gaining any weight. After a few sessions, out of desperation, I calmly asked if anyone else was getting the milk. "Yes!" the mom said, "I also give it to my older child, so he can be nice and healthy, too." Although many women tandem nurse (meaning nurse their older child as well as their newborn), this is not a good idea if the infant is having any kind of weight gain problems. In this instance, the newborn baby should take priority, and all the milk should go to the newborn until the weight gain problem is resolved!

Weaning

I sometimes define weaning as "a permanent solution to a temporary problem." Mothers can be so exhausted or frustrated after childbirth that they throw in the towel at the first sign of trouble. One of the problems here is that moms often have "weaning remorse," and then want to fully relactate. It's not that it can't be done, it's that it would have been easier to fix the primary problem. If you're considering weaning, please get some good advice on how to proceed.

At any rate, should you decide to wean at any time, it should be done gradually and naturally. Optimally, in a perfect world, it should take two to six weeks or longer and be "baby-led." Baby-led means that the baby decides when to stop breastfeeding. If this is not something that resonates with you and you want to start sooner, pull out all the stops. Wear a gently supportive bra, even to bed at night, take Sudafed, suck peppermint Altoids to excess, and wear cabbage in your bra morning, noon, and night. You should also take Advil, 600 mg, every six hours for a couple of days. Empty the breasts a bit if they're getting too hard and be careful not to get mastitis (a breast infection). Optimally, decrease by one feeding every five to seven days or so until your milk supply is dry. It's also wise to let a lactation consultant guide you through this process.

You can also wean using a breastpump and feeding the baby a bottle. Just cut out pumping sessions one at a time, like you would feedings. Moms with babies who tend to bite sometimes prefer this. This allows you to control the exact duration of feedings and suction at specific intervals. It's also much easier than pulling baby off in the middle of a feed because you don't want the breast to be too stimulated.

There are lots of books written on weaning, so I won't try to explain exactly how it should be done within the context of this book. Just be prepared for an emotional loss when weaning and compensate with extra cuddling.

Nursing Strike! Union, Union, Union!!!!

All of a sudden, and often without any warning, your baby can strike from feeding at the breast. If baby is under one year, be careful not to interpret this as baby-led weaning. So, what's a mother to do while the baby is picketing with his union sign? This may last anywhere from one feeding to a month (rare). Causes can be environmental or physical. Here are some things to try when trying to cross the picket line:

- Wait 10-15 minutes and offer the breast again while skin-to-skin.
- Pump your breasts (as often as baby was feeding) to maintain your milk supply, and give baby breastmilk in a bottle. Repeat as necessary.
- Wait him out, but don't get engorged to the point of pain and suffering for you or the baby.

If you've changed your perfume, deodorant, toothpaste, or lotion, the baby might not recognize you. I had one such mom (during a home visit), shower and put on her old perfume. The baby ate like he hadn't seen her all day! The little guy was starving. "Mom, thank heavens you're back! Some other lady with weird smelling perfume tried to feed me while you were gone."

Phantom Feed (aka Dream Feed) - When the baby is asleep in your arms at night, while it's dark and quiet, slip a breast out of your bra, express some milk onto your nipple, and bring him to the breast. The baby will start to nurse in his sleep and forget all about that silly picketing.

This is another one of those times when lactation consultants can really earn their keep!

Types of Breastpumps: Get Yourself a Helmet and a Seatbelt

I think it's worth it to buy breastpumps from a lactation consultant who will sit down and explain how to put them together and use them. You may or may not spend a few extra dollars, but if you do, it's likely money and time well spent. Especially if you plan on going back to work or need to work on increasing your supply, you will be spending a lot of time with your pump, and you need one that is effective and efficient for you.

Basically there are three types of pumps: rental pumps (or hospital-grade), expensive purchasable pumps, and inexpensive hand-held pumps.

Rental pumps are closest to approximating a baby's suck. You rent them by the week or month, but buy your own kit (personal pieces that attach to the breast). Kits are around $50 and rentals are about $75 a month. They're worth every penny. Rental pumps are great if you're having difficulties or are returning to work. Several companies make these pumps: Ameda (Elite), Hygeia, and Medela.

One popular brand, the Medela Symphony, has a two-phase expression. This means you get a full two minutes of nipple tickling (stimulation) before it goes to the second letdown phase. I did have one mother of seven tell me to "knock off the foreplay and get the milk out" when I was demonstrating the tickling stimulation phase. Having said that, most mothers really like it.

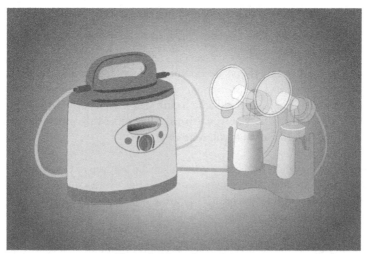

Figure 2.6 Symphony Pump

Midrange Expensive Purchasable Pumps (meaning $150-400) are pumps that you buy after your milk supply is established and flowing well. Around the third or fourth month, you may get tired of renting and just need something to cart to a part-time job. If you have oversupply issues, then you can use this pump sooner. If you're not going to breastfeed close to the full year, you don't need one of these. You really shouldn't transfer them to another owner, so you'll just end up discarding it. Ameda makes the Purely Yours, while Medela makes the Pump-in-Style or Freestyle.

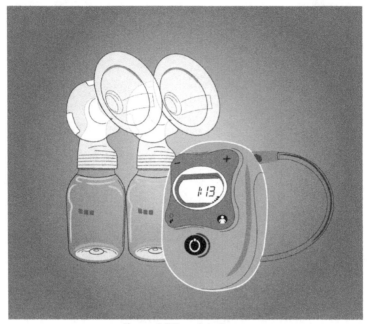

Figure 2.7 Freestyle Pump

Inexpensive Hand-held Purchasable Pumps (aka toys). This is for a mother who only wants to pump a couple times a week. You can get tennis elbow squeezing or pulling the lever. These also fill in for the Orthodox Jewish moms who do not use powered equipment on the Sabbath. Avent Isis, Medela Harmony, and Ameda One-Hand are three popular brands.

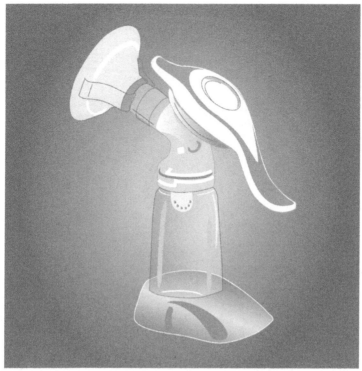

Figure 2.8 Manual Pump

For all of these pumps, 20-30 minutes is usually the magic number to be double pumping (both breasts at the same time). In my experience, pumping longer doesn't do anything but cause nipple soreness. Some moms find that pumping two minutes or so after their second letdown works well, too.

Moms have individual milk output patterns, and triggering at least two milk ejections during a pumping will drain the average mother's breasts as fully as her baby will (Mohrbacher, 2010). Of course, it then stands to reason that triggering three to four milk ejections will drain her breasts more fully (Mohrbacher, 2010). This is helpful in instances of trying to increase production or making up for fewer feedings that day.

If, while pumping, your nipple starts to bleed, lower the suction, and then stop. Moms often resort to pumping when they have sore nipples and the trauma is already established. I only mention this because it's a frequent question. Don't toss out the milk. Allow the blood (which is heavier then milk) to sink to the bottom, pour off the good milk on top and discard the bloody milk. If the baby swallows the blood, since it is an irritant in the stomach, he may vomit it back up. When breastfeeding, you usually can't know if the baby has been swallowing bloody milk, and it can be pretty unsettling to see your infant spit it back up. Keep in mind, the blood came from you and your baby is not bleeding. Call your lactation consultant or healthcare provider if this happens.

Look Ma, No Hands!

With a bustier-type bra that will hold the breastpump pieces to your breasts throughout the pumping session, you can have your hands free to do other things while pumping. You can eat your lunch, get on your laptop, or take a much-needed nap. (Make sure you have a timer on, for obvious reasons!)

One of the current hands-free products I like is a pumping bra from Simple Wishes (2010). It looks like a pink bra top with two openings (criss-crossed panels) in the front to hold the funnels of the breastpump to your chest. You can use the straps if you're large-breasted to give you a bit more support.

Another choice is to cut small slits in an old sports bra and use that as your hands-free pumping bra.

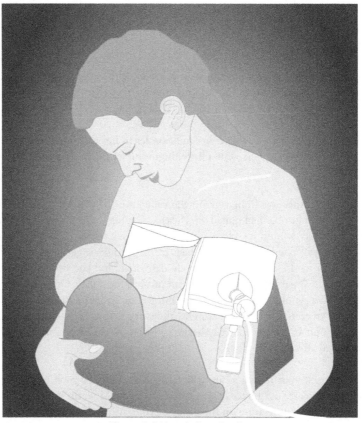

Figure 2.9 Hands-Free Bustier

Express Yourself – Literally - Hand Expression

There are some moms that only need a little bit of expressed milk from time to time, and they prefer to hand express it. It can be quite effective, but I wouldn't recommend it for long-term needs like going back to work.

Hand expression, although like a little elliptical exercise for the hands and breasts, is very effective, inexpensive, and can produce results worthy of your labor. There are many techniques and videos available on the Internet. One only needs to google "hand expression of breastmilk." My favorite video demonstration can be found at http://newborns.stanford.edu/Breastfeeding/HandExpression.html.

Got More? Time to Store

Now that you've pumped it, what should you do with it? According to the American Academy of Pediatrics, freshly expressed milk is good for six to eight hours at room temperature (meaning up to 77 degrees). If you know you're not going to use it within that time period, then freeze it. It's good in the fridge for five days, good in a household freezer (with a separate door) for three to six months (keep it way in the back), and good in a deep freezer (one of those big square chests that is only for freezing) for 6-12 months.

When you're working and putting it in a cooler with refreezeable ice packs, it's good for 24 hours, but make sure it's not any warmer than 39 degrees by having the cooler pack touching the milk (CDC, 2010).

I had one mom pump and forget her milk cooler in her car overnight. It was still good the next morning (she kept a little thermometer in the cooler), and she was very happy.

A not-so-great story was from a mom who called me as I was writing this book to report that her plumber had pulled out the electric plug to her deep freezer because he needed to get behind it. He forgot to plug it back in, and she didn't discover it for two days. She had stored 300 bags of breastmilk to get her baby through her return to work. The milk was totally defrosted, and she wept for days. The plumber said "What's the big deal? You can just use formula." One has to wonder if the plumber would have said the same thing if mom had 300 pounds of prime beef in her freezer. The happy ending to the story is that we calculated she only needed 12 ounces for her first day back. She was able to successfully pump that amount, and all was well.

If you've frozen your milk and are wondering how long it's good when you take it out of the freezer, 24 hours is my answer. You should warm it in a pan of hot water, check the temperature on the inside of your arm by sprinkling a few drops, and then feed it. You cannot refreeze it once it's been defrosted and thawed. Never microwave breast milk — overheating destroys valuable nutrients and "hot spots" can scald your baby's mouth.

What Type of Container to Use

The best options for storing human milk (La Leche League International, 2010):

- Glass or hard-sided plastic containers with well-fitting tops

- Containers not made with the controversial chemical bisphenol A (BPA)

- Containers which have been washed in hot, soapy water, rinsed well, and allowed to air-dry before use

- Freezer milk bags that are designed for storing human milk

Disposable bottle liners or plastic bags are not recommended. With these, the risk of contamination is greater. Bags are less durable and tend to leak, and some types of plastic may destroy nutrients in milk.

When you are storing milk, put only 60 to 120 ml (two to four ounces) in the container (the amount your baby is likely to eat in a single feeding) to avoid waste. Do not fill the containers to the top - leave an inch of space to allow the milk to expand as it freezes. Mark the date on the storage container. Include your baby's name on the label if your baby is in a daycare setting.

Chapter 3

Issues with the Mechanics of Breastfeeding or Trouble, Trouble Right Here in River City

Below you'll find a quick interpretation of some common breastfeeding problems to give you a very basic understanding of these maladies. For more detailed information, try either www.kellymom.com or www.llli.org.

Plugged Ducts

A plugged duct (aka milk duct or lobe) will feel like a small knot that is under the surface of the skin. It may wax and wane, but you can definitely feel it. It results from a duct not draining well. Perhaps you've had breast surgery or an injury to that breast. It also may have started from holding your thumb over the duct area while breastfeeding, allowing the milk to clog, or it might have been caused by a restrictive bra. Your breast(s) may feel warm, and you may have flu-like symptoms. Regardless of the cause or the symptoms, this can be a precursor to the next problem: mastitis.

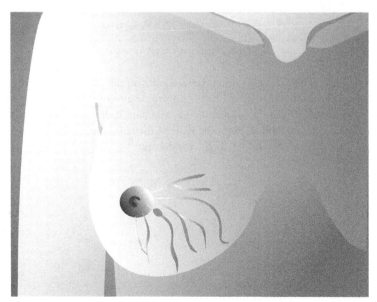

Figure 3.1 Plugged Duct

Treatment for plugged ducts involve application of warm compresses before either feeding or pumping, and cold compresses to the area after feeding or pumping. Try to point the baby's chin in the direction of the plug. Picture your breast with a clock superimposed over the front. If the plug is at 12:00 noon, place the baby's chin at the top of the breast by using the illustrated hold.

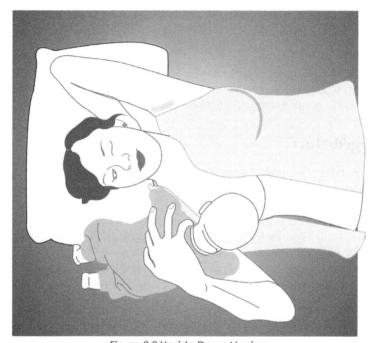

Figure 3.2 Upside Down Nursing

The chin area is where all the action takes place. If you can gently massage the plug and push it toward the nipple, it'll help. You should also try 600 mg of ibuprofen every six hours to decrease the inflammation and curtail the pain. Lots of bed rest is key (I know, it is so hard to find time with a little baby, but it's important), as is keeping the breast empty and latching baby deeply.

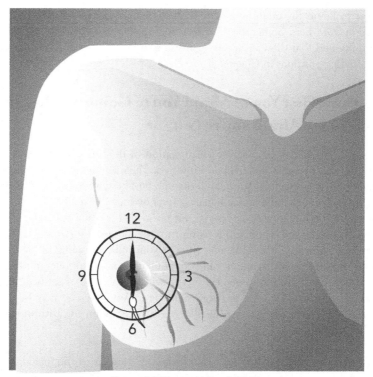

Figure 3.3 Plugged Duct Clock

When the plug comes out, you may see the baby gag. If you've pumped it out, don't be surprised to see a long, stringy, white strand of milk. Picture the skin that forms over milk on the stove—it is like that. It's not harmful to the baby, other than perhaps a bit of gagging.

A tip for preventing chronic plugged ducts is to take Lecithin tablets, which are made from soy. You should take 1200 mg (one tablet) three to four times a day. You can stay on this product the entire time you're breastfeeding.
Note: If you have an oversupply, you should not use the Lecithin.

A final tip: If you are trying the above tips and the plug still persists for more than a few days, see a lactation consultant or your physician. I had a friend die in her 50s from breast cancer, which her doctor had initially diagnosed as an unresolved plugged duct. Plugged ducts should go away.

In my practice, I had one mom come in to see me with a plug at the top of her breast (12:00 o'clock). I told her to breastfeed with the baby's chin in the direction of the plug, and I'd be right back into the room in about ten minutes. When I returned, she was holding the baby upside down by his feet! She was hanging his head over the front of the breast. The poor baby's head was beet-red. I had meant for her to lie on the examining table with the baby's feet going in the opposite direction from hers. Sometimes, I forget how specific I need to be when I give directions, and that this can be very confusing for moms. See the illustrations of breastfeeding positions in Chapter 1, Figures 1.1 to 1.7.

Mastitis: First You're Afraid You're Going To Die, and Then You're Afraid You're Not

Mastitis is miserable and involves inflammation of the breast. It may be caused by a plug that becomes inflamed and infected. There are many types of mastitis, and they are all miserable. You may feel some flu-like symptoms and like you've been hit by a truck! You'll probably have a fever over 102.5. You'll have an area on your breast (on one usually, but maybe on both) that is really red and extremely hard and tender. Don't confuse this with primary engorgement (around day three) where you can get only a slight milk fever as your milk is coming in. When you suspect mastitis, then it's time to call your primary care practitioner, midwife, or OB. If you're not allergic to penicillin, you will probably be prescribed 500 mg of Dicloxacillin four times a day for 10-14 days. Anything else may be under-treatment. If you're allergic to penicillin, get a prescription for azithromycin or clindamycin.

Major predictors for mastitis and causes for mastitis are varied and include: stress, plugged ducts, a tight bra, nipple pain, cracked nipples, difficulty taking the breast, restricted breastfeeding, overabundant milk production, consistent pressure on the breast, baby sleeping for longer stretches at a time, ineffective milk expression, too-rapid weaning, uneven breast drainage, history of mastitis with a previous child, milk appearing thicker than normal, and a nipple that looks misshapen after a feed (Mohrbacher, 2010).

Keep in mind that the milk is still good when you have mastitis, but it may decrease in quantity. It can also cause the milk to taste salty. Keep feeding your baby or pumping, even though you feel sick. You can lie on the couch, feeling sick as a dog, and let your partner bring you the baby to feed.

If you do not get proper, prompt treatment, mastitis can become an abscess. This is a walled-off area of pus inside the breast that will need to be incised and drained or aspirated in order to get relief.

Thrush the Magic Dragon

Because there's always yin to the yang, the antibiotics which cure mastitis can set you up for thrush. Some mothers that were GBS-positive (Group B Streptococcus) at the time of delivery will develop thrush from the antibiotics they are given prior to and during delivery. Some women get repeated cases of thrush, even if they haven't taken antibiotics.

Thrush is yeast that naturally occurs in your digestive system, but can appear in an imbalanced way, either in your baby's mouth or on your nipples, and will likely spread from mother to baby and from baby to mother. It's an eco-system. Your nipples may become very sore while breastfeeding and will appear to have a glaze over the top. You can also have breast pain, which may indicate that you have thrush syndrome. This is when you need treatment for both you and the baby. The baby should either be on oral Mycostatin or Diflucan, and you should be on both oral Diflucan and APNO (All Purpose Nipple Cream). Get online and search for "thrush syndrome," "antibiotic treatment," and "breastfeeding." You should also start taking a good probiotic (the "good bacteria" that live in our gut, to chase out the yeast) like Florastor, two capsules twice a day. You can also give your baby some probiotic powder by putting it on your nipples before you feed him. Culturelle can be a good choice. Check out your local natural food stores for a good selection of probiotics for adults and children. If your child has a sensitivity to milk, be aware that many probiotics contain milk products, but there are some that do not.

Thrush can be difficult to get rid of, so in addition to taking oral and topical medications, there are other steps you can take to try to keep thrush at bay. You can apply Gentian Violet on your nipples and coat the baby's mouth with it. It is a treatment that has been around for ages, and it can be found over-the-counter at some stores. It is extremely messy and stains skin for several days. You can apply Vaseline to the baby's lips prior to application in his mouth to avoid purple lips, although I have seen many an interesting dark-purple mouthed Goth-baby, donning the telltale signs of Gentian Violet, and it is kind of cute. There have been some studies indicating that overuse of Gentian Violet can have negative side effects, so consider using it one time in the baby's mouth and two times the same week on your nipples. Remember that if you breastfeed after the application to your nipples, your Goth-baby will reemerge.

Because yeast thrives on moisture, avoid breast pads if possible, but if you must wear them, use the disposable ones and change them after each feeding. Diet also plays a role in yeast overgrowth. You should try to avoid consuming a lot of sugars (natural and artificial) and refined carbs. (I know, I know, you're already in pain from the thrush, and now this crazy lady is telling you to cut out sweets, too!) Also, it is important to try not to re-infect yourself while you are treating both yourself and the baby. Wash all of your bras, towels, and clothes in hot water with bleach. Dry in a hot dryer. Boil for 20 minutes or disinfect your pump parts or any pacifiers daily.

Breast Shape

Widely spaced breasts (more than 1½ inches) and tubular (aka Hypoplastic Breasts) or cone-shaped breasts may have problems with milk production. If your breasts look like this, you may not have enough glandular tissue to support breastfeeding. This is not the end of your world. Many mothers can and do exclusively breastfeed. This is written as a heads-up. You can still breastfeed and wear a supplemental nursing system to bond with your baby, even if you're supply does not allow you to open a Dairy Queen.

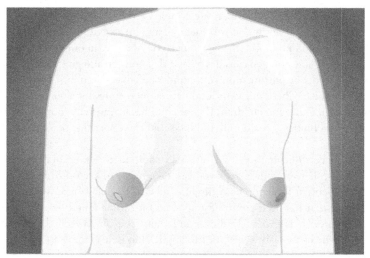

Figure 3.4 Hypoplastic or Tubular Breasts

Flat Nipples and Inverted Nipples: Whose Idea Was It for our Breasts to be Boneless?

When you squeeze the darker area around the nipple (the areola), your nipple should evert (stick out further). If your nipple inverts (puckers or dimples in), you may have an inverted nipple. If it neither goes in or out, it's flat.

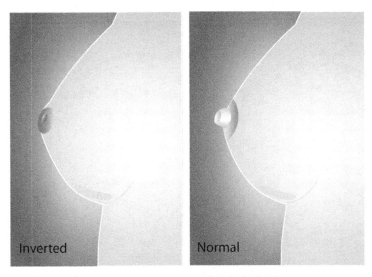

Figure 3.5 Inverted and Everted Nipples

Since the baby needs something poking into his mouth to stimulate the suck spot, both flat and inverted nipples suck (pun intended). Relax, there's a tool called a nipple shield, which looks like a miniature silicone sombrero. You can wet the perimeter of the shield, or rub some lanolin around the perimeter, and paste it over your nipple. The baby gets stimulation to the roof of his mouth and starts to suck. The shield has lots of holes at the end for the milk to come through.

Make sure the nipple shield is a "contact shield," meaning one made with a contour at the top, so the baby can bring his nose right up to the breast. Also, check the size (in millimeters). Extra small is 16 mm, 20 mm is a bit larger, and 24 mm is the largest. The Medela website is a nice resource to continue reading about nipple shields and their proper use (Medela, 2010). You should try to remove the shield, if possible, during the nursing session. Since it blunts the proper stimulation, you may want to rent a hospital-grade pump to compensate with some additional "sucking" time. You WILL want to wean baby off of it as soon as possible. Lactation consultants are very helpful with this.

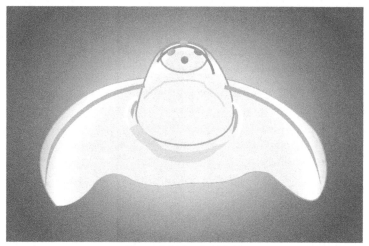

Figure 3.6 Nipple Shield

Large Nipples

Sometimes, nipples are very big and baby's mouths are very small. I think I've seen the largest breasts in the world feed a little preemie baby and it worked! (I guess nobody told the baby.)

If this is a serious problem, you can always pump until the baby grows into the breasts. If you do decide to pump, remember to buy bigger flanges (27, 30, OR 36 mm), so your nipples aren't getting squeezed into the regular (read small) diameter flange hole. Pumping shouldn't feel like you're sharpening a pencil.

The Case of the Missing Nipple

Once in my office, during a nursing teaching session, I asked a mother to "switch breasts." She explained she couldn't because she didn't "have a nipple" on the other side. She was born and raised in Germany and had been shaving her legs with a straight razor. While in the shower, as she was bending over, the razor came up and cut the nipple off! YEOWWWWW!

Tight Lingual Frenulum: Something You Never Had to Think About Until Now

Under the baby's tongue, right in the center, is a type of fleshy string called a lingual frenulum. It can sometimes be a little too short and tight, and can cause incredibly sore nipples for moms. If your breast tissue is soft and pliable, your baby may still be able to feed easily. If your breast tissue is more firm and taut, the same degree of tongue-tie may cause more of a struggle (Mohrbacher, 2010).

Some babies have a frenulum that is so tight it causes the tip of the tongue to come into a heart shape when the baby cries. This is colloquially referred to as being "tongue-tied." The frenulum in this case needs to be clipped by a doctor for two main reasons. First, it will make breastfeeding a whole lot easier because the baby will be able to stick his tongue out properly when suckling. The second reason is much further down the road. Some children have such an extremely short frenulum that when they say words with "th" in them (try saying this, that, these, those), they can't stick their tongues out over the lower gums. If this tight lingual frenulum is discovered in an older child, perhaps by a speech therapist, the procedure is a much bigger ordeal, requiring general anesthesia. If it's addressed as a newborn, the procedure will cause one small drop of blood after a local topical anesthetic. The baby can immediately come right back to the breast and, man oh man, will you feel the improvement.

An eight-year-old patient with a lisp came into our office for a physical exam. Since he had been with our practice his entire life, I became nervous about who might have missed his tongue-tie during his first couple weeks of life. After flipping back through eight years of notes, I realized that I was one of the practitioners that had seen him and had charted that the parents did not want their baby subjected to this "barbaric" procedure. I felt bad for him because he told me the kids at school made fun of his lisp. He subsequently underwent the surgery at eight years of age, under general anesthesia. I remember him telling me how his tongue felt huge, like it completely filled his mouth and took up every bit of space. I thought about how strange it must have been to release the tether, and then not know what to do with a wild tongue. It took two years of speech therapy to change his lisp.

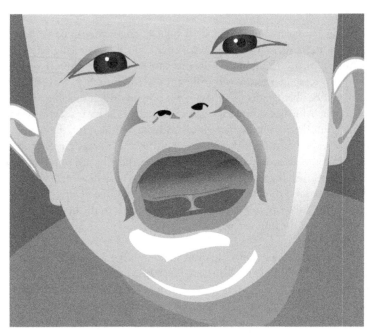

Figure 3.7 Tight Lingual Frenulum

Chapter 4

Artificial Breastmilk
(AKA Formula or Non-Human Milk)

Going to an AA Meeting

So, I realize that a lactation consultant giving formula to a breastfeeding mom is like an AA meeting gone bad: you go to the meeting and the moderator says, "Here's the twelve steps buddy, but if they don't work out, here's a six pack of Bud Light for you!" (Or formula, as the case may be). Sometimes, though, formula may be necessary.

I always feel bad when I have to recommend formula to a mom who has clearly told me her goals are to breastfeed. I only do this under one circumstance: when a baby has lost more than 10% of his body weight and mom's milk is not in yet, in which case I recommend formula as part of a greater plan to get the baby's weight up. To improve the milk supply, I typically get the mom double pumping (see "The Draconian Schedule," Chapter 1), and sometimes have the partner finger feeding the breastmilk (with a periodontal syringe to prevent nipple confusion). Only when we've discussed the benefits of this schedule, do I hand over some of our cheesy samples of free formula. Keep in mind that formula is not rat poison.

Types of Formula or What's Baby's Point of Reference for Flavor Anyway, a Good Chardonnay?

Formulas are the only food regulated by the FDA. They all have to meet specific standards to be sold in the U.S. Therefore, all formula brands are nutritionally sound when moms are unable or unwilling to breastfeed.

There are basically three types (bases) of formula: cows' milk, soy, and pre-digested proteins.

Cows' Milk Formulas are the basic ones handed out in hospital nurseries to mothers who say that they're breastfeeding (just kidding). Cows' milk has evolved for baby cows, but it's available in vast quantity and can be modified to become an acceptable formula base. Cows grow at a rate 47 times that of humans, so their milk contains a large amount of protein. This can be very difficult for babies to digest, although most do quite well on it.

If you notice that when you're feeding a cows' milk formula, your baby suddenly develops a rough, red, itchy rash all over, this might be a protein allergy. Also, the baby might have blood in his stool. Stay alert. I ask moms who are breastfeeding to try stopping all dairy products when their breastfed babies develop this rash.

Soy Formulas are an alternative to cows' milk formula when babies develop an allergy. Soy is the largest plant protein available, and babies can also do quite well on it their first year. Vegan parents usually prefer soy as an option.

Pre-Digested Protein Formulas use cows' milk proteins, which have been broken down into very small pieces. These formulas are marketed as hypoallergenic formulas for babies with colic or gas. Generally, I think these formulas are best for all breastfed babies. Yes, they smell bad, they stain, and they are very expensive, but they also tend to agree with babies the best.

All formulas are recognized in the body as a solid food. They sit in the belly like a Thanksgiving turkey dinner and can sometimes cause the baby to sleep for longer periods of time. This is not the reason they should be used. Breastmilk may only last for about 90 minutes in the tummy, but it keeps the baby on a more natural rhythm and is correlated with a lower incidence of SIDS. Babies also stool easier on breastmilk diets.

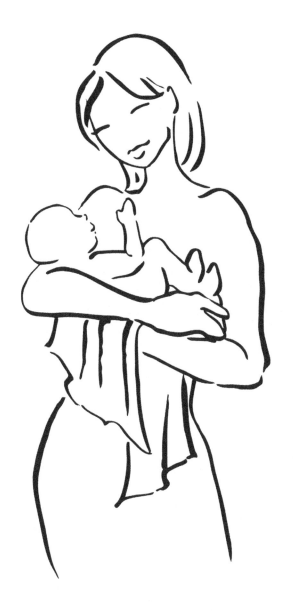

Part II

TAKING CARE OF YOURSELF AND YOUR BABY

Chapter 5

Calming

Crying Baby & Comfort Care—Back to Basics

Remember that it is OK for babies to cry, as long as you offer some type of comfort when you hear them. It's not OK for a baby to cry and cry, and be ignored. Some babies cry more than others, just like some people talk or yell more than others. It is their way of communicating. When a baby cries, it does not mean you're a bad mother. It does not mean that your mom or Aunt Mabel would know exactly what to do, and you just don't. The process of figuring out why your baby cries is a language that you and he are creating together. He cries because he is upset about something—sometimes he doesn't even know why. And you respond by calmly and confidently picking him up and reassuring him that you are there. Just by being calm and holding him, you are telling him that you will be there when he cries and when he doesn't, that the world is OK. So take a deep breath…Ahhhh. You two will figure this out together.

Sometimes, it is helpful to start out with the fundamentals. If your baby cries, pick him up. Plain and simple. Clinical studies show that mothers who responded promptly to their babies had babies that cried less (St. James-Roberts, Bowyer, Varghese, & Sawdon, 1994). A newborn does not realize that you and he are two different people. He's been floating around in your tummy for 10 months and doesn't know anything else. The baby wants to be with you, on you, next to you… you get the idea. I often wondered why women weren't born with a kangaroo pouch. Wouldn't that make life easy? Since you can't spoil (what does that word mean anyway?) a baby less than six months or so (no matter what your mother-in-law tells you), it's perfectly fine to hold them as much as you want. In fact, it's preferable!

Babies cry because they are overfed formula, underfed, or sometimes because they are over stimulated. It was pretty Zen in the womb—dark and quiet. Re-create that for him. Try nursing (or bottle feeding), rocking, and/or temporarily swaddling the baby—all are womb-like activities. Remember, that whatever method of calming you try, it's important to give it a little time to work; otherwise, you might overwhelm the baby and make the crying worse. If all else fails, try switching to someone else holding the baby. Your baby might sense your frustration, which could be making things worse.

Chamomile Tea or Fennel Tea (Gripe Water)

Exclusive breastfeeding, meaning without any supplements of any kind, is always best. If you want to drink these things yourself, now that's an idea!

Sleeping With Baby

Your baby wants to be and should be near you, with you, on you, and next to you. Have you ever been to a farm? Where are all the baby animals? Under their mothers, on their mothers, suckling their mothers, etc. I'm not saying that humans are farm animals, but we are mammals, and our babies want to be with us. Is that such a crime? Read about Secure Attachment...go ahead, Google it. Do you want a kid that grabs your leg and won't let go when you're trying to drop him off at daycare? Then stop pushing him away and trying to get him to sleep alone in his own room by himself all night. I do believe you need some time for yourself, as well, but maybe not for the first couple of weeks. It goes fast; trust me. I know each tired day feels like an eternity, but you can do this!

As far as keeping the baby in bed with you throughout the entire night (aka bedsharing), that's a pretty controversial subject. There's a lower incidence of SIDS when babies are put on their backs to sleep. There are potential risks involved with every sleep setting, whether it's a separate crib or bassinet in their own room, or in the parent's bed or co-sleeper. Researchers have concluded that the co-sleeper (or side-car) appears to be the best of all the sleep options (Mohrbacher, 2010).

Introducing Your Baby to the Concept of Sleeping on his Own: Ritualize the Bedtime

There's nothing funny about a baby who doesn't seem to want to sleep or parents that could fall asleep in their soup. It's not safe. It's very important to establish day and night patterns for everyone's sanity. Here are some of my own suggestions for bedtime, when you feel it's time to get more organization in your days and nights:

- The room should be blackout dark. This may mean buying blackout shades or even taping something over the windows to make it pitch black.
- Get a white noise machine, not the trendy one with the cute cricket sounds or the babbling brook, but the one that sounds like the radio in between stations. Make it fairly loud. Not enough to burst the eardrums, but loud enough to block out all the fun stuff that will be going on outside.
- Remove all the stimulating toys from the crib. This includes gyms and mirrors attached to the side of the crib, mobiles, and stuffed animals. Who can go to sleep while lying in the middle of Disneyland? You can

leave in one lovey of sorts after three months, just make sure it's not fluffy.

- After 12-16 weeks of age, TRY putting your baby down while he's still awake. You can still rock him and sing, but if you put him to sleep that way, when he wakes up he'll need you to soothe him again. What you've taught him is that the only way he can fall asleep is through you, so he'll cry when he wakes up, wanting you to soothe him back to sleep. Having said this, do go back into his room when he needs you. Parents ask me this question all the time. Should I go back? Yes. The baby needs to know that he is OK and not alone. It's important to note that the AAP recommends babies sleep in the moms' room for the first six months. The policy states that this should be done in a "separate but proximate sleeping environment," (p. 1252) meaning crib, bassinet, or cradle (American Academy of Pediatrics Task Force on Sudden Infant Death Syndrome, 2005).

Make Him Sleep Make Him Sleep Make Him Sleep!!!

Stroller rides in the house and driving around the neighborhood are two tried and true mechanisms when all else fails. Put your baby in a stroller and find a nice little "bump" someplace, i.e., a place where the carpet overlies the wooden floor or under a doorway where you have that nice, small strip of wood. Slowly push and pull the carriage back and forth rhythmically over the bump. You can also try a walk inside or outside (weather permitting) with baby in a sling. I always did my housework wearing my daughter. I was able to feel like I was accomplishing something, and she was happy as a clam!

You can also put your baby in his car seat and take a little ride around town. I did this with both of my children, and would coordinate naptime this way. I used to take a book with me, so if they fell asleep, I could pull over someplace safe and just read. One day, sleep overtook me, and I woke to find a nice policeman knocking on my window, asking if I was okay!

My daughter was always a horrible sleeper. She didn't sleep through the night once until she was two years old. I didn't have anyone to teach me any of these tricks! I was so exhausted that I'd lie down with her in the afternoon, trying to get us both some sleep. I remember one afternoon in particular, when she woke up before me. She was prying my eyelids open saying, "All done sleepies, Mommy!" and then again at twice the volume, "All done sleepies!" Babies never seem to let you nap when you need one.

For different resources on sleep and calming, I personally like the video, "Happiest Baby on the Block" (for the visual learners among us) to help parents learn to swaddle (don't like the early use of the pacifier) (Karp, 2003). There are plenty of really impressive books on breastfeeding that I've mentioned in the resource section. Find an author that speaks to your heart. Remember, take away what you think is valuable and helpful for YOUR baby and you; leave the rest.

Chapter 6

Coping With Motherhood

Your Body (or at Least It Used to Be)

Following the birth of your child, your body doesn't look or feel exactly like it used to, which can make you a bit weary or depressed. Let's see, you're bleeding (a lot!), your vagina may be swollen and bruised, your perineum (the area between vagina and anus) may be very sore (from episiotomy, stretching, or tearing), your belly may still be big and covered with stretch marks, and your breasts are big and may be leaking (see Chapter 2). Yuck.

Although you may be delighted with the lovely new being you've produced, your appearance and pain may, very understandably, leave you feeling downright crappy. Have faith, though, that like the process of getting to know your baby, the process of getting your body back will work, but it might take some time and effort. Oh, avoid those tabloid pictures of celebrities who are back to a size zero only three weeks after pregnancy—unless you have a cadre of personal trainers, nannies, cooks, and personal assistants —your recovery will be less dramatic and will take more time.

More Blood Than a Horror Movie

You may be shocked by the amount of blood emanating from you after birth. That and the fashionable fishnet underwear supplied by the hospital are the lovely little tidbits that friends and family neglected to tell you about the birth experience. Postpartum bleeding is called *Lochia*. Lochia is your body's way of expelling placental tissue, excess mucus, and blood after giving birth. It may feel like it will never end, but rest assured it will probably only last for a few weeks. It feels like having a very, very heavy period, but you should not wear tampons, just wear pads.

The blood may be accompanied by uterine cramping that may feel worse while you nurse. The cramping is a result of your uterus contracting to get back to a much smaller (but not original pre-pregnancy) size. While the blood and cramping may make life feel a bit miserable, they are both a normal part of recovery. The cramping should reassure you that you're making the nursing hormones prolactin and oxytocin, which, in turn, are responsible for milk supply and letdown reflexes.

Welcome to Your Temporary New Vagina: Cavernous, Bruised, & Battered

Following a vaginal birth, your vagina may be swollen and bruised, and your perineum (the area between vagina and anus) may be very sore (from episiotomy, stretching, or tearing). Also, the whole area may look different. Yes, feel free to go ahead and look. Get a mirror if you want.

The swelling should go down within days, and the muscle tone should return more quickly if you do Kegels. Kegels can help regain pelvic floor muscle tone and help with incontinence issues. Your vagina will not look like a cave forever, but keep your partner from spelunking in there until after your first postpartum physician checkup.

The soreness of your vagina and perineum is also normal during the initial postpartum period. Those weird hospital-issued sitz baths really do help with healing. Also, short of straddling an ice sculpture, the hospital-issued or homemade ice-packs are best for soothing the pain in that whole area.

Weight Loss and Body Image

Yes, you may still look pregnant after birth. You may even get the horrifying, "When are you due?" questions for weeks or months after the birth of your child. You may have curves where there were no curves before. Chances are you will lose much or all of the weight you gained over the first year that follows the birth of your child. If you had a *linea negra* (black line) or stretch marks during pregnancy—those too will fade over time.

Try to take care of your body, as well as your baby's—exercising, eating well, and breastfeeding all help hasten the weight loss process. Treat yourself to some pampering activities away from the baby to make you feel better about yourself—a pedicure, a manicure, or a new hairstyle can do wonders for your self-esteem.

Factor in that you probably haven't really felt like making love during the last few weeks, and that can just add insult to injury when it comes to your primary relationship. Remember, women tend to be much more sensitive and critical about their appearance than men are. Keep in mind that most partners aren't looking at the fact that you gained some weight. They're looking at how beautiful the mother of their child is. Again, give yourself some time and be kind to yourself. You won't walk out of the hospital wearing your skinny jeans. It took you ten months to get here; it'll take you about the same amount of time to get back.

When I was pregnant with my second child, I gained (a ridiculous!) 78 pounds. During pregnancy, I was always hungry, so I was always eating. My grandmother told me if I had a craving I didn't satisfy, I'd give birth to a baby that had his mouth hanging open all the time. (I know you've seen kids that look like this.) I thought it was a good excuse to eat and eat and eat. At my last OB visit, the doctor casually mentioned that if I didn't stop eating, I'd have to "deliver at Sea World." In the end, I dropped all the weight (but not necessarily gaining back the tone). With an 18-month-old and a newborn, I ate most of my meals off the highchair while breastfeeding. Not glamorous, but good multi-tasking and highly effective for weight loss!

Postpartum Depression vs. Baby Blues

This section is both the easiest and the most difficult to write. Easiest, because I had a terrible case and can tell you first-hand what it's like; most difficult because it was so damn painful.

There aren't always perfect indicators for what constitutes postpartum depression in a mother. Having said that, I now believe I know it when I see it and understand there are some common themes.

Inflammation has recently been identified as the risk factor for postpartum depression that underlies all other risk factors (Kendall-Tackett, 2007). When inflammation is combined with other risk factors (sleep disturbances, stress, physical pain, nipple pain, etc.), cells are released from the immune system causing physical inflammation and depression (Kendall-Tackett, 2007; Mohrbacher, 2010).

What's important to remember is that moms are usually home from the hospital after the first day or two. Unless she and her partner have prepared for getting some help at home, it can be a very lonely, stressful, and difficult time. She is left alone to feed herself, teach herself to breastfeed, and recover from birth (Kendall-Tackett, 2010). Is it any wonder moms get bummed out?

Baby Blues are common, as more than half of new mothers have them. The symptoms are reminiscent of PMS: irritability, crying, anxiety, impatience, and lashing out at those you love...you get the idea. Compound this with the new demands of motherhood and exhaustion, and you have the perfect storm. I tell moms this usually gets better after the first month or so.

But what if these symptoms DON'T get better? If these feelings become more consistent and severe, it's probably become PPD (postpartum depression). Approximately one in five mothers will have PPD. Not all will get treatment.

It's very difficult from the practitioner's standpoint to help these moms because very often they (the moms) truly don't know they're depressed. They channel their depression into other venues, and that's why it can look different depending on the mother/baby couple. Some (but not all) common feelings of PPD are:

- Increase or loss of appetite
- Difficulty sleeping (despite being exhausted)
- Feeling restless
- Not enjoying things that previously brought you pleasure
- Feelings of guilt
- Either lack of interest in your baby or being totally obsessed with every little detail

Red flags warranting an immediate call to the obstetrician or primary care provider include (Kendall-Tackett, 2009):

- Thoughts of suicide
- Substance abuse
- Days without sleeping
- Quick weight loss
- Lack of normal grooming
- Inability to get out of bed

I had a colleague tell me once that if I (as the clinician) felt depressed after a visit with a mother/baby couple, I could pretty much count on the mom having PPD. That advice has served me well.

For me, when I was a new mom, I felt totally overwhelmed by the responsibility of caring for my babies. I wasn't secure about my parenting skills and was eternally sleep deprived. I just was too embarrassed to say that to anyone. It was the mid 80's, and nobody so much as hinted to me what I was feeling in my heart. Obviously, I got through it, and perhaps that's why I'm writing this book 27 years later. I'd like to help other women avoid enduring the same fate.

If you even think you might be depressed, you probably are. Recognize how common this mood disorder is and ask for help. There are therapists who can really make a difference. There are medications (safe while breastfeeding) that can substantially help improve your mood and, thereby, your life situation. It's also been proven that moderate exercise (meaning 40 minutes three times a week) can be as effective as medications in treating PPD (Blumenthal et al., 2007). To take it a step further and actually offer you a solid recommendation, 20-30 minutes of exercise two to three times a week is suggested for moderate depression, and 45-60 minutes of exercise three to five times per week is recommended for major depression (Kendall-Tackett, 2009).

Other treatments for PPD include psychotherapy, herbal medications, light therapy, and taking Omega 3-fatty acids. These are all covered in depth in the websites noted below.

If you'd like to explore this topic in depth, I recommend reading *The Hidden Feelings of Motherhood: Coping with Stress, Depression, and Burnout* by Kathleen A. Kendall-Tackett (2005).

For those among us who need an instant knowledge fix, there are incredibly helpful handouts on both www.BreastfeedingMadeSimple.com and www.UppitySciencechick.com.

Parents, especially mothers, desperately need social support, which isn't always available (or affordable). Family members, friends, neighbors, support groups, church groups, moms' groups, La Leche League meetings, etc., are all ways of getting this kind of support.

One other final thought and very important reason moms should seek treatment for PPD is that, in addition to affecting her life and relationships, a mother's depression can also affect her baby. So, in making life easier and better for herself, she also makes life easier and better for baby.

Baby Come Back - You Can Blame It All on Me

PPD Storytime: You know that I'd have to have a funny story for this serious situation.

I remember watching my husband get ready to go to work and wanting to recreate the Psycho shower scene. I hated him for leaving me alone with two little ones. He was getting dressed-up, putting on aftershave, thinking about what restaurant he would be dining in for lunch, and walking out to meet other freshly showered, happy people. I could barely manage brushed teeth and a ponytail. I wish we would have talked about it more. Not that there was necessarily anything we could have done differently, but because it caused problems. Now, in reflection, I can see it all so clearly. At the time, a friend suggested a therapist.

Fast forward to a young, pretty therapist-thing telling me I should go back to work (I was so exhausted, I couldn't even shower most days), and I should make special, little fun times and meals for my husband (she had to be kidding! That's insane! Why just last night I ate a sandwich on the floor of the bathroom with one baby on the potty and the other on my breast). She just didn't seem to GET IT. She didn't understand what it was like to be a mother! She was hitting raw nerves here. She was making the monster mad! I came to the conclusion she was NOT the right therapist for me. I asked her if she had any children of her own.

"No, but that doesn't matter as I fully understand all the issues of motherhood." (WHAT? Not a chance that you possibly can fathom what the hell my life, or any other mother's life, is like...mumble, mumble...my mind reeled). I left therapy that night. I remember thinking, "LOSER," as my engorged breasts let down milk because I had been away from the baby too long.

Fast forward three years. I'm standing in the hallway of the pediatrician's office (working), as I see this woman come down the hall, crying her eyes out and being physically supported by her husband and mother. Guess who it was? YEP... So, I said to her, "See? I told you it was unbelievably hard!" That was the last time she came to our office! And I'm glad...I hope she had a good therapist!

Witching Hours

Let's face it! By 4:00-7:00 o'clock at night, we've all had it with the day. That's why we have happy hour in this country. During these hours (which I call the witching hours), babies cluster feed about every hour on the hour. Your baby is getting ready for his big sleep. Like a camel getting ready to cross the desert, he's tanking up on food.

Older people occasionally experience a phenomenon called "Sundowning." I remember working in a nursing home where the residents showed a dramatic increase in agitation and confusion in the late afternoon and evening. One theory for this behavior is that they become so overloaded and stressed by all that goes on during the day they can't adequately process it all. One reason for this is declining or limited cognitive abilities. By evening, these residents were so over-stimulated they reacted in the only way people with limited options for communications can react. Some cried, some hollered, and others became disoriented and wandered.

Infants can do something pretty similar, reacting with utmost crankiness and a feeding frenzy in response to their own daylong stimulation. Unfortunately, that frenzy comes at the end of your long day, too.

If you've ever been a stay-at-home mom, you know that last hour when you are waiting for your partner to come home takes forever. The child has ramped up all of their annoying behaviors, and you are so done by this point that you are watching the clock furiously. And God help you if your partner is late. I remember screaming at my husband one night when he had said he'd be home by 6:00, and it was already 6:10!! The baby had had it, too, probably with ME.

So, what do you do? You can try to have a late afternoon/evening routine that works for your kid(s) and you. For me, it used to be the 4:00 p.m. walk, followed by the 5:00 p.m. early kid dinner, followed by the 5:45-6:00 p.m. bath, preferably performed by Dad. By 6:30 we'd (Dad would) be reading a story, and by 7:00 p.m., it was lights out. Establish a ritual of your own by finding something that works for you! A ritual helps your baby recognize that he is heading to bedtime, too, so he (and consequently you) can wind down.

Also, your partner should, of course, help with the kids when (s)he gets home. Often, the point of marital strife comes when your partner wants a break when (s)he gets home from work, and all you want is a break from the kids. It is hard for everyone, and a compromise needs to be made. Perhaps your partner can take a few minutes to unwind and relax, and then it's your turn.

Also, it may be hard for you to switch gears from playing with the kids all day to being with your adult partner. I remember when two kids under two equaled rough days for me. When Adam (my first, practice baby) was eight months old, I was pregnant again (OK, so one night I wasn't that tired...it happens). Anyway, I remember spending most of my days looking at these cute little pinhead babies all day long. One evening, when my husband came home from work and kissed me hello, all I could say to him was, "GOSH, YOU'RE HEAD IS HUGE!"

Whiskey, Wine, Beer, and Other Coping Strategies

A common question I get asked is, "Can I have some beer or wine with my dinner if I am breastfeeding?" Absolutely. What do you think the mamas in Rome, Italy, are doing tonight? First, you will want to wait until baby is at least a month old before drinking ANY alcohol. Then just remember to take it easy. Don't drink regularly (meaning every night) and not more than one drink at a time. It's always a good idea to drink AND eat some food at the same time. Alcohol peaks in your breastmilk in 30-60 minutes (InfantRisk Center, 2010). For each normal drink you ingest, you should wait about two hours per drink. If you wait two hours per drink, the amount of alcohol in your breastmilk will be much less.

Although baby has a liver, it's new and smaller than yours. You can keep baby from having to process the alcohol by pre-pumping (prior to drinking) for the next feeding or pumping and dumping (down the drain) if you prefer.

You can purchase strips of paper (Milkscreen) that tell you for sure when the alcohol is totally out of your breastmilk. I don't think you need these for that small, occasional drink, though.

Chapter 7

Mom How-To's

Pacifiers Suck!

When you're trying to teach your baby how to breastfeed properly, why trick them? How would you like it if you announced you were hungry, and someone handed you a stick of gum? What part of hungry didn't you understand? The bottom line is that during the first few weeks, it's almost impossible to differentiate a feeding cue from a true sucking cue. It might be better to err on the side of caution and try feeding first. I know the baby will take the pacifier, but he may get frustrated because he hopes milk will come out.

Having said that, there are special cases where a pacifier can be beneficial, but only after the baby is about a month old and breastfeeding is firmly established. Sucking can help to relieve stress. It's difficult being a baby. Think about it, babies are limited to crying to communicate. They poop and pee in their diapers all day long, they get gas, they have occasional reflux (heartburn), and people are in their faces saying, "gootchie gootchie goo." The baby can't curse, pour a glass of wine, or take it out on someone else. So, your little one is left to suck away his stress. If you have a barf baby (a baby that spits up a lot), giving a pacifier after a meal may help.

So, why is it important to wait to use the pacifier until the baby's about a month old and only after your milk supply is established? Studies show that mothers who use pacifiers regularly will breastfeed fewer times per day (Mohrbacher, 2010). This translates into both a lower milk supply and not enough food for baby.

It should be noted that pacifiers are only for infants. I've seen two-year-olds sucking on pacifiers, but extended use of a pacifier can interrupt speech development and cause dental problems.

I once had a dad in my practice honestly ask me if it was OK to put two small pieces of duct-tape over the edges of the pacifier because it kept falling out of the baby's mouth. Umm, in a word, NO! Why do men always want to fix everything with duct-tape anyway?

Tummy Time

Although babies need to sleep on their backs to prevent SIDS, they should have 30 minutes of SUPERVISED tummy time each day, starting from the first week or two. Tummy time helps increase babies' motor skills—it helps them to learn to sit up, roll over, pull-up to standing, and, eventually, it helps them develop the muscles and habits necessary for crawling. If you need to, you can break the half-hour a day into segments. Sometimes, it helps to have a thumb stuck into the mouth when on the tummy.

Your baby's favorite place to sleep is on your chest—it is a wonderful place to be. Studies show that if your baby is lying on you (either to eat or snuggle), it will regulate his pulse, heartbeat, respirations, etc. However, chest time spent fairly vertical does not count as "tummy time," anymore than adult push-ups on the side of the wall count as real push-ups—it is not enough of a workout. It does count as tummy time when you are fairly flat on your back and baby is on top of you.

Boxing Gloves and Other Sporting Equipment Should Be Left off Your Baby

I was guilty of this 25 years ago, so I'm not looking down my nose at you, but please keep mittens off your baby's hands. Sometimes, parents even improvise and put socks over the baby's hands. When parents try to explain, "Her nails are too long," I ask, "Do you wear gloves if you don't have time to file your nails?" After some nervous laughter, it starts to make sense. Babies are learning so very much about their world when they're born. I believe the sense of touch is an important way to learn about their environment.

If you were to take a newborn baby and blindfold him for the first two weeks, the sense of sight would never develop, so it follows depriving the baby of touch would be equally as detrimental. The baby needs to experience his world—that mom's breasts are soft and warm, that dad's arms are hairier than moms (hopefully), and that there are many different and exciting textures in the world.

Often parents say, "But I'm scared to cut the baby's nails. I might take a finger off." Good point. Instead, use a soft paper emery board and file at right angles until you're feeling more comfortable.

Why do Belly Button Cleaning? I'm Stumped!

Although some hospitals will tell you not to clean the umbilical stump, I think it's OK if you do. The stump needs to dry up and fall off. Don't be squeamish about it. You can't pull it off by moving it North, South, East and West to gently get some rubbing alcohol around the base. It will also smell a lot better! You really don't need to call the doctor if there's a bit of blood around it; just clean it again at the point where you see the dried blood. If you decide to just tidy up, cleaning the stump once a day is usually enough. Having said this, you don't HAVE to do it.

Occasionally, the cord will fall off and leave a small glistening yellow piece of tissue in the center. This is called an umbilical granuloma, which is a fancy name for the remaining living tissue. When you go to the pediatrician, they may cauterize it with silver nitrate. Cauterizing doesn't hurt the baby. Silver nitrate sticks are also commonly used for dogs' and cats' nails that have been cut too short. It acts as a sealant. The procedure will temporarily cause a small dark brown or black smudge, but it can be cleaned out in about a week. It doesn't hurt, either.

Rub A Dub Dub - Three Tricks in the Tub

While we're on the subject of cleaning, bathing your infant should not be a scary experience. To wash his hair in the early days, hold his head over the sink and use some baby shampoo, rinsing with a cup of warm water. A sponge bath will do until the cord falls off and you can submerge your baby's body. Run a Q-tip around the top of the ears (don't try to clean out the ear canal), and use a washcloth behind the ears. You've heard the expression "wet behind the ears?" That's because babies lie on their backs and drool. The drool dries and becomes crusty, so clean behind the baby's ears on a daily basis. A very gentle cleanser, like Cetaphil Lotion Soap, is best for all the baby's delicate areas. If an area gets a bit red, add some healing ointment, like Vaseline or Aquaphor. If the skin cracks and is open to infection, call baby's healthcare practitioner.

Baths are fun for babies when the cord is off and they can be submerged. It reminds them of returning to the womb. Make sure the temperature is warm, and that the baby is in the mood (read: not currently hungry, exhausted, or recently awakened from a nap). Bath time is some of the only exercise and recreation the baby gets, and it can be a regular part of the bedtime ritual.

Girl Baths

Girl baths should involve spreading and cleaning the labia. Spread the lips of the labia with your left forefingers. With a warmly water-moistened cloth, wipe once on the right side (top to bottom). Find a different area of the cloth and repeat on the left side. Finish up by finding another clean area of the cloth and wiping once down the middle. It will become second nature. You don't need to "excavate" all of the cheesy white coating here, just clean out any fecal matter.

Boy Baths (Circumcised)

Baths with circumcised boys should involve keeping the foreskin back where it belongs. After a couple weeks, make sure the foreskin does not turn into a penile adhesion—this occurs after circumcision when the middle, pinker part of the penis rejoins the outside skin at the base. Call your healthcare provider if your son has an adhesion. He or she can teach you how to care for an adhesion, and make sure that you are very, very gentle in this endeavor!

Boy Baths (Uncircumcised)

If your son is not circumcised, then no extra cleaning of the penis is required in the newborn phase. The urinary meatus (the opening where the urine comes out) should be rinsed off during a bath, however. Watch for redness or swelling if your baby is not circumcised.

How Long Has Itzbeen Since We Changed the Diaper?

It's OK to rely on a tracking system for the first week or so. Some parents need a way to ensure their babies are getting fed and changed, and they simply don't trust their tired brains to do the mental tracking. The good news is that there are lots of ways to keep track of everything that's going on with, or in, the baby. I've seen every method from Excel spreadsheets to hash marks on dad's hands.

There are even gadgets to help you keep track of how long it's been (get it?) since you've either changed a diaper, fed baby, or put baby down for a nap. You can use something as simple as a piece of paper with the date at the top. You get the idea.

Whatever tracking method you use should be discontinued when the baby is up to birth weight, and you feel like you're seeing a recognizable pattern. Unless the baby is not gaining an ounce a day, there really is no reason to bring this journal into the pediatric office or to continue to use it.

Just keep in mind that for the next couple months, there should never be a time when you go more than six hours or so without changing a diaper. I always tell parents, "Watch the baby, not the clock."

Chapter 8

Your Baby's Health

The Hospital

I have a few thoughts on what's important if you're delivering at a hospital. I always share the following in my prenatal and breastfeeding classes.

If you are going to breastfeed, deliver at a hospital that's designated "Baby Friendly." The Baby Friendly Hospital Initiative (BFHI, 1991) was launched by WHO and UNICEF in 1991, following the Innocenti Declaration of 1990. The BFHI designation ensures that, if breastfeeding, you and your baby will get the best possible care. Breastfeeding is promoted, supported, and protected in these hospitals. This will make your first days a lot easier.

If it's not possible to deliver at a hospital that has the BFHI designation, request that your baby:

- Not have a pacifier
- Not be given any supplementation unless medically indicated
- Be breastfed in the first hour of life
- Room-in with mom
- Be fed on demand

For successful breastfeeding, you should not accept anything from a formula company. I don't believe (even if their gifts are for breastfeeding moms) that they generally give you the best feeding information. You'd be amazed at how tempting it is to just pop a top off the formula bottle in a frustrating moment. Without the temptation, you may be more inspired to find other solutions.

Most hospitals have lactation consultants (LCs) available, as well as discharge classes. Plan on attending one, and plan on securing some resources for your first days at home, just in case. Ask the LC to observe your latch whether you think you need it or not. By nipping (no pun intended) it in the bud, it might save you from painful latch problems later.

Hopefully, you've already chosen a Pediatrician or Nurse Practitioner. He or she might come to the hospital where you'll be delivering. Make sure your practitioner knows you plan to breastfeed exclusively and supports your wishes.

Also, calling a local Lactation Consultant (LC) in your early days at home is not a bad idea. She or he can tell you about her services and availability, and a conversation early on helps by just knowing you have someone familiar to call.

The Revenge of Cabin Fever or Find Your Takeout Menus

Babies are born pretty tough and remain that way for about the first 30 days. They have all of your antibodies on board because they were grown within your body. Breastfeeding continues to give some protection, but until they're fully vaccinated, they just aren't ready for prime time! Be aware that from the fall to the spring, babies are at risk of getting the highly contagious Respiratory Syncytial Virus (commonly known as RSV). This virus can exhibit itself like a common cold in adults and older children, but for babies, it is much more serious. It may make your baby very sick and in need of an inpatient hospital stay. This means that it's not such a great idea to take the baby to a restaurant, grocery store, or the gym's baby room.

During any season really, it is not a good idea to go to a lot of public places during the first couple of months. One exception is to keep your baby in a sling, so others aren't touching him. There are times when being cooped up in the house can be pretty suffocating for moms and dads.

Keep the visitors to a minimum, or at least limit who handles the baby. Remember, engage in lots of hand washing, and do not allow visitors (big or little) with sniffly, snorfly noses to be around the baby. I've seen lots of babies catch colds from different sources, and it's really not pretty. Remembering that all babies for the first few months are obligate nose breathers, you can imagine what happens when *one nostril gets* totally clogged. If you think you already lie in bed and listen for them to breathe, try lying there listening to the chronic snorting. Congested babies are unable to nurse well. When they have a stuffy nose, babies will nurse like a swimmer...head down to nurse, then head up to breathe. If your baby is really not nursing because of a cold, it is time to call your healthcare practitioner.

Wait until the baby has gotten a little bigger and stronger before you subject him to the germs of strangers. You can still go for glorious stroller walks and car rides and have healthy visitors to the house. (Watch the children of healthy visitors.) It's even OK to go to a friend's house with your baby. Just don't overdo it. In summary, it's just not worth it for a couple hours in a restaurant.

Baby al Fresco

Strange places can be as unsettling to your baby as familiar places can be boring. For that reason, I advocate taking a new baby into every room of your house on his first couple of days home. That way, there are no strange places within your home. However, babies can get cabin fever just like we can. It gets pretty boring staying indoors all the time looking at you. As previously mentioned, be wary of taking your baby to public places with lots of people in the first couple of months. That said, though, just a walk outside may be the stimulation both you and your baby need. If you go outside, there is the excitement of lights, sights, sounds, and smells to stimulate and refresh your baby's (and your) senses.

Keep in mind that your baby must be dressed appropriately. This means if it's winter, use a snowsuit, hat, socks, and blanket, and keep the outing short. If it's summer, dress lightly, but avoid direct sunlight. A good rule is that babies need one more layer on their bodies than we have. If you're comfortable in a short-sleeved shirt, put baby in a short sleeve shirt plus a light sweater. If you have your winter parka on, use baby's snowsuit plus a blanket.

One well-meaning father in my practice tried to get his baby some fresh air by parking his 4-month-old in the yard, with the stroller top partially raised. The baby was well shaded until the sun moved, and the father didn't notice. After the baby had been asleep in the sun for well over an hour, he suffered a severe sunburn on half of his face.

If you are going to take your baby out, you need to protect him against the sun. It is important to cover your baby with protective clothing and a sun hat. Try to keep him in the shade or make shade with a stroller hood or an umbrella. Plan to go out in the early morning or late afternoon, when there is less exposure to ultraviolet radiation. We used to think you should not put sunscreen on babies younger than six months old. Now, the American Academy of Pediatrics (AAP) suggests small amounts can be used on an infant younger than six months after you have taken the other precautions mentioned above. There are so many "baby" sunscreens though; it may seem difficult to choose which one to use.

When To Call the Doctor (Errr...Healthcare Provider)

Babies don't have the same reserves we have, so they get sick faster. The good news is that they also get better faster.

When my daughter was in intensive care as an infant, I heard the most useful advice I've ever heard from a doctor. Erin was acting well, despite her working diagnosis (meaning what they thought was wrong with her). The doctor looked at me and said "Sick babies LOOK sick." I know this sounds simplistic, but it really does make sense. When a baby is really sick, they usually won't eat, sleep, or make normal eye contact.

Here's a short list of some red flags to look for that require a call to your healthcare provider:

- Rectal temperature of 100.4 or above when your baby is under four months of age, and especially under two months of age, even if you think he looks OK, or you "know" it's his older sister's cold

- Not eating as much or as often as usual

- Poor or no eye contact

- No social smile, providing they're old enough to smile, usually by two months of age

- Sleeping way too much or way too little

- Inconsolable crying

- Grunting instead of breathing

- Color change of the baby's skin

- Vomiting and/or diarrhea lasting for more than a day

- Very little urine (babies should urinate at least every six hours)

Help Me, Help You

In order for your baby to get the most out of your visits to your pediatric healthcare provider, the relationship between you, as parents, and your provider needs to be a real collaborative partnership. Your provider's responsibilities are to make sure your baby has appropriate medical care. We make the determination as to the best course of action after doing a thorough examination, and hearing from you and your child about the details and history of any medical issues. In order to give an accurate diagnosis and treatment plan, you need to provide as much and as accurate information as possible. Your provider needs to really respect and listen to you and your child, respond appropriately to your concerns, and come up with a plan that works. Sometimes, the best plan does not involve any major medical intervention. Parents and their provider need to have an open exchange of ideas. Don't be intimidated by a lab coat or a stethoscope. We're working for you. Like Tom Cruise said to Cuba Gooding, Jr. in *Jerry Maguire*, "HELP ME, HELP YOU!"

As pediatric health providers, we have dedicated our lives to helping your children. Most of us love what we do. Sometimes, though, parents get very frustrated with us. To be honest, most frustrations have to do with parents' unrealistic expectations of us and parents' not-always-correct ideas about pediatric health. A better understanding of where we're coming from may make your visits more pleasant. I hope to clarify the following misunderstandings:

1. Frustrating and miserable symptoms in your child do not always require medical intervention. We know that colds can be miserable for your child. Your child has a runny, yucky nose, he's coughing, he's having trouble sleeping, he's cranky, he's clearly uncomfortable, and he's crying. And crying. And crying... He's miserable and so are you. You're frustrated because you've tried everything you can think of and you want your provider to do something for him. Fix it. Now. Here comes the tough part—we can't fix it. If it's been diagnosed as a viral upper respiratory infection, there is no cure and no medicine. Antibiotics do not work for viruses. Your provider may call your child's cold a "viral rhino sinusitis" or a "viral upper respiratory infection," but what your child has is a cold.

We use elaborate terms for simple illnesses to validate your feelings of frustration and let you know we are not downplaying your concerns. Your child will get over his cold, or at least feel better, in a week or so. That said, of course, you can bring your child to the office to make sure it is a cold and not an ear infection. Oh, saline and hugs are your friends. Spray saline into your child's nose at regular intervals and provide copious amounts of lovin' to your sniffly, cranky little one. Everyone needs their mommy when they are sick, and you may just be the best medicine after all.

2. We don't always have the answer. Sometimes, we can't pinpoint the exact cause of your child's illness. There is no such thing as a perfect parent, and there is no such thing as a perfect healthcare provider. We know a great many things, and, most times, we can come up with an accurate diagnosis. We do have access to a large arsenal of resources on diagnostics. Ultimately, though, we may not come up with an exact answer. We can do thorough exams, ask you lots of questions, and compare your child's symptoms to our knowledge of diagnostic criteria for illnesses. We can also compare your child's symptoms to symptoms of other children we have seen with known diagnoses, or we can ask a colleague with more experience. We can order tests and rule out lots of potential causes. In the end, though, we just may not know what is causing your child's illness. We can recommend specific courses of action that may (or may not) help, tell you definitively what it's NOT, or refer you to a specialist. But again, we may not have a definitive diagnosis for you. Just please don't freak out because we tell you we don't know something. It does not mean that we are not good practitioners—in fact, it is the good ones that will admit to such a thing. What is important, though, is that we communicate with you our thoughts, and that we work *with* you to find a course of action that is the best for you and your child.

3. Too many cooks spoil the broth. Dr. Google, your list serve, your mother, and your friend from the playgroup are NOT the licensed healthcare practitioner you've chosen to take care of your child. Please do not come into our offices demanding certain tests be performed because you are sure you know what is wrong. We do want to partner with you and hear your thoughts, though. You have picked

your healthcare provider for a reason; please let us do our job. We have extensive education and experience, we know your child's medical history, and we truly care about your child's well-being. We are more knowledgeable than your non-provider friends and relatives, and, yes, we are even more knowledgeable than the Internet. Many Internet sites are just opinions from patients, and even the ones written by doctors are biased because many are sponsored sites. An interested party, such as a pharmaceutical or other special-interest group, pays for sponsored sites. If you want the most thoroughly thought out and objective treatment plan, it is not fair to you or your child to rely on advice by the well-meaning non-medical community.

OK, thank you for listening!

Hiccups and Snorty Noses

All babies are obligate nose-breathers for the first few months. They cannot breathe out of their mouths. They can't pick their noses, blow their noses, or do that guy-in-the-shower-thing. Buy a small bottle of baby salt water nose-drops: Lil Noses, Na-sal, Ocean, Baby Ayr, and other cutsie names for the exact same thing - 0.9% sodium chloride. Don't use the one that's been up your nose. Also, do NOT use contact lens solution because of all the preservatives.

Gastroesophageal Reflux Disease (G.E.R.D.) Vs. Colic, or Why Has My Baby Turned Into Oscar the Grouch?

The dreaded colic is usually defined as unexplained crying (read: you're fed, changed, held, and nothing's poking you, and you're still crying?) for up to a few hours once or twice a day. Colic starts around three weeks of age and tapers off by 8-12 weeks. Some parents try gripe water or Mylicon at this point. Either is fine, but they probably treat parents more than babies.

Sometimes, babies can become unreasonably cranky. They develop hiccups, nasal congestion, and spit up after most meals. Although all babies have these symptoms occasionally, babies with G.E.R.D. have symptoms that are truly "over the top." Parents frequently ask me what they're doing wrong and tell me that they and their infants simply don't sleep. There is a definite desperation when parents come in to see me for this visit. These babies are usually gaining weight normally, or even better than expected, but they're miserable.

The cause of these symptoms is the leakage of food and stomach acid back into the lower esophageal sphincter, resulting in feelings of heartburn. In order to find relief and self-comfort, babies naturally want to suck. If the sucking takes place on a breast or bottle of formula, overfeeding can exacerbate the reflux. We often recommend keeping babies upright for 15-30 minutes after a feed. Car seats are no longer recommended, as they tend to jack-knife the baby's legs at a 60 degree angle and can exacerbate the reflux. I really like teaching parents what I call the "colic-hold," which is designed to keep the baby upright and puts a tiny bit of pressure on the left side of baby's body.

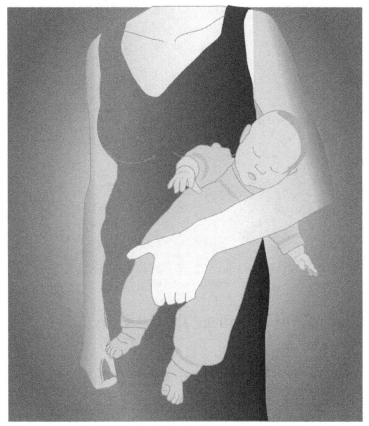
Figure 8.1 Colic Hold

Think about how you feel after gorging on Thanksgiving dinner. It can be very difficult to determine if your baby is truly hungry or just needs a pacifier. You can TRY the pacifier after a feed (once the baby is above birth weight), and if they're not hungry, they should relax. If they are hungry, they'll probably spit it out and cry for something with milk behind it.

Not all babies spit up or projectile vomit when they have reflux, so the diagnosis can be difficult to make. The regurgitation continuum starts with crankiness and hiccups, and escalates up through noisy burps, gagging, seeming to re-chew or re-swallow food, and spitting up. Then it continues to a stage where you might want to feed your baby on a tarp and hose him off afterwards. Keep in mind that there is such a thing as the "happy spitter." These babies are the "feed on a tarp" types, but aren't cranky about it, and, in fact, may smile at the laundry they've generated.

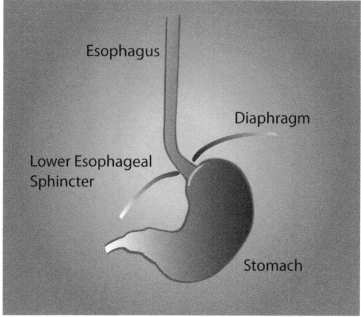

Figure 8.2 GERD

Barfing and Other College Tricks - Party Like the Romans

Some babies, like some Roman aristocracy, overeat, vomit, and eat again. Herein lies the difficulty of trying to figure out if it's reflux (the weak sphincter), overeating, or both. You simply have to get to know your baby, as there's no easy answer.

To determine approximately how many ounces a baby can eat by bottle, divide their body weight by two and subtract one. If the baby weighs 7 lbs, half is 3.5. Subtract one. The baby can eat 2.5 ounces. Remember, this is his maximum stomach capacity. Most of us don't eat to maximum stomach capacity, so this is just a rough estimate. If you're solely breastfeeding, you'll have to wing it--breasts don't have those measuring lines on them. Look for the baby being content and having adequate output.

For babies who are frequently spitting up, you can watch the baby for signs of fullness and burp frequently. You can also cut them off a few minutes before they're finished and see if they'll take a pacifier for the last two minutes. Most practitioners won't treat these kids medically, but will recommend the precautions below.

I had a little girl in my practice that vomited faithfully after each feeding. Her mother either took her out to the yard to feed or put a plastic tarp under her high chair in the kitchen. She swore if it continued she'd begin to use the garden hose to clean her up. Thankfully, by one year, the problem resolved. Since she loved to eat, weight gain was great. There wasn't any discomfort after eating, so it wasn't a problem. As the gastroenterologist said, "It's more of a laundry problem than a medical problem."

One trick to keeping reflux at bay is to keep the baby upright for 15-30 minutes after eating. Avoid changing the diaper immediately after feeding as well. Have your baby sleep on a gentle incline by raising the head of the crib or bassinet mattress and placing a folded towel under it. Some parents choose a wedge-shaped sleep positioner. You can also walk around with your baby in the colic hold (see Figure 8.1).

Cow's milk in mom's diet or in the baby's formula can, in some less common cases, exacerbate reflux. Try supplementing cow's milk with Alimentum (if you must use a formula while breastfeeding) or completely eliminate milk products, like yogurt, cheese, ice cream, milk in coffee or cereal, from your diet. You can also add a good probiotic, like Culturelle, every day.

If your baby is one of the cranky ones with reflux, see your pediatrician or a pediatric gastroenterologist for a prescription for Zantac. If Zantac doesn't hold back the symptoms, your baby may be prescribed Prevacid.

Some additional thoughts on causes of reflux are all easy to understand. If you are breastfeeding and have an oversupply or your milk lets down with a gush, it's like having someone put a garden hose in your mouth while turning on the spigot. It's hard to keep up. If this happens, there are many different ways to control it. You can buy and use a nipple shield (the silicone miniature sombrero described earlier). This will act as a governor and only allow some of the milk through the holes in the top.

Remember to remove the nipple shield immediately after the letdown, so you don't decrease your milk supply. If you have an incredible milk supply, you can use one breast per feed to insure baby gets lots of hindmilk. Generally, hind milk comes out later in a feeding and is richer (has a higher fat content). Foremilk satisfies thirst; hindmilk satisfies appetite. Another way to control your abundant milk supply is to recline during the feed, so the baby feels like he's drinking out of a water fountain, rather than a garden hose.

Jaundice is Like the Golden Curtain Rising

Jaundice is caused by a build-up of broken down red blood cells. When the umbilical cord is cut, the baby's body yells, "Hey, way too many red blood cells here." Jaundice is analogous to ashes in the hearth after a good log burns. The baby's tiny liver is about the size of the end of your finger and is panting like a dog to filter the blood. Be patient. In order to decrease the concentration of bilirubin (the end-product of red blood cell destruction), you have to increase the food in the body to increase output at the other end. Babies have to poop it out, so to speak. You can see the amber color in the diapers (known as bili-stools). Terrific.

Jaundice can also be caused by blood incompatibility between the baby and the mother. We perform a test called a "Coombs test." When babies are positive, they're at a greater risk for developing jaundice. Whatever the cause, whatever the result, if the baby is jaundiced, you do the same thing - feed, feed, feed. Our motto to avoid this situation is "Breastfeed early and often!"

In earlier years, we asked you to put your partially undressed (diapered) baby in the window (behind the glass) and let natural sunlight do the work of hospital bili-lights. We have discovered that this does not work, and, therefore, no longer recommend it.

If your doctor or nurse practitioner is concerned about the degree of your baby's jaundice, she may send you to a lab to have the bilirubin level checked. They will prick your baby's heel and squeeze the blood out to test the level. You'll probably feel really sorry for your baby when his heel is being pricked for tests every day, but it is always better to be safe. Hospitals will also use a TCB, which stands for transcutaneous bilirubinometer. This meter can check a bilirubin level by holding it to the baby's skin and is not painful for babies.

The level of bilirubin that can cause problems depends on how old and how developed the baby is. If the bilirubin is above a certain threshold, you may have to go back to the hospital for 24 hours or so. If the hospital is detecting a problem with bilirubin very early in the baby's life (the first 24 to 48 hours), that's a greater concern.

Bilirubin levels should be solidly under 20, but if it's creeping up to 17 or 18 and the baby is not gaining weight and not breastfeeding well, your healthcare provider may jump into a short-lived action plan of your own version of the Draconian schedule or may add formula. Each case must be addressed on an individual basis.

As a parent, don't be afraid to ask your practitioner about checking the blood levels. They'll decide, based on many different factors, if this is necessary. Keep in mind, we like to see things resolve naturally when we can, rather than have baby readmitted to the hospital.

As jaundice goes away, it improves from the feet up. The last things to improve are the eyes. Babies can stay jaundiced for several weeks. It's important to know that for most newborns, jaundice is temporary and usually resolves on its own.

Chapter 9

The End Result: Poop (and Pee).
Let's Not Spend a Lot of Time Here.

Input, Throughput, and Output

I frequently get the question "How do I know if my baby is getting enough to eat?" The answer is easy. If the baby is satisfied after feedings, there are plenty of wet and poopy diapers, and your child is gaining weight, your baby is eating enough. This isn't rocket science, but it's also not an exact science. You'll want to continue to check the baby's weight periodically to make sure he's gaining a consistent one ounce per day for that first month or so.

Ideally, you want to have one wet diaper and one meconium stool on day one of life, two on day two...up to day six to seven, when six or more wet diapers a day and approximately three to four stools is appropriate. Just make sure by day four or five that the stools are turning yellow and seedy.

It can be challenging to decide when poopy diapers are also wet diapers. If that's something you really need to ascertain, you can wrap your boy's penis lightly in a tissue. In girls, it's a bit easier because of anatomy; you know what's coming out the front and the back.

Autumnal Colors of Poop

The question of poop color is a very common one, and it often causes great concern in parents. My answer never varies—any of the autumnal colors are fine. Breast stools are very yellow, like mustard, bilirubin stools are more of a dark amber color, and formula stools are browner.

Sometimes, stools can be green. This is not a cause for alarm if the baby is happy and gaining weight appropriately. Consistently green stools (sometimes with mucus) may indicate sensitivity to a substance he is getting from mom's milk (medications or diet) or that he is not getting sufficient hindmilk (fattier milk) during a feeding.

The number one offender from mom's diet causing green stools is usually dairy products: milk, yogurt, cheese and puddings. Other foods that can cause green stools are soy, seafood, peanuts, chocolate, citrus, wheat, eggs, and corn.

A white stool or a lot of blood in the stool is not normal. Mucus or blood in the stools can be a sign of a sensitivity or allergy and should be reported to your baby's healthcare provider.

Poop Etiquette

Please don't bring dirty diapers to the pediatrician's office unless you really need to show us something important, like a gallon of blood. As a matter of protocol, we really don't care to stare a turd in the face. Seriously! This is not The Little Emperor! Your description will be more than fine.

Also, please carry out what you carry in (take dirty diapers home with you, for those of you not familiar with "the camping rule"). There's nothing worse than having to work in an exam room with the smell of dirty diapers haunting your day. When a parent asks, "Where does this go?" I answer, "Home with you." Note: Bring a plastic bag with you wherever you go. It's just the polite thing to do.

Red Alert, Red Alert - Houston, We Have a Problem

Blood in the diaper is one reason for lots of calls to the pediatrician. These babies should all be seen by a healthcare practitioner, but it's usually one of two things and neither is a dire emergency.

The first reason there could be blood in the stool is if the baby has an anal fissure. Since formula is recognized in the body as a solid food, it can make babies constipated. When pushing out a dry, hard stool, the baby's bottom can get an anal fissure, which is almost like a vaginal tear during labor—the skin in the anus can split and blood appears. The blood gets streaked onto the stool. This situation usually resolves without a lot of intervention. A little petroleum jelly right around the sphincter can make the baby more comfortable. Many moms get hemorrhoids during pregnancy and can empathize with their baby's painful situation.

The second reason may be the baby is hypersensitive to a protein food (i.e., cows' milk protein), either from formula (soy or cows' milk) or through your breastmilk (mom's diet), that does not agree with the baby, and the problem is coming from higher up in the gut. Again, your healthcare provider will help determine why your baby has blood in his diaper. The office may perform a stool guaiac test, which will give evidence of whether the blood is frank (you can see it) and/or occult (not visible to the naked eye). This test gives us a clearer idea of what is going on and how to treat it.

Constipation - Who Gives a Crap?

This is really a two-part answer. In the newborn period, especially during the first week, there are fairly uniform guidelines on how often babies should stool. The Academy of Breastfeeding Medicine (2007) considers indicators of adequate mother's milk intake to be yellow stools by day five and three to four stools per day by day four of life.

Constipation means hard, infrequent stools. After six weeks of age, totally breastfed babies might not necessarily poop once a day, but when they do, it's usually soft. If babies are happy and comfortable and stool every few days or even once a week, with a nice soft stool, AND they're gaining weight, then you don't have a problem.

Yes, if it's going in, it will come out, but keep in mind that if formula has been introduced, they may start to have a problem with fewer stools AND harder consistency.

If the baby is crying, grunting, and passing hard "rabbit turds" (meaning small pellets), infrequently, then you probably have a problem.

During the baby phase, older than two months, you can try a liquid glycerin suppository, which looks like a miniature enema. This can often irritate the rectum and lubricate the anal sphincter enough to make the passage of stool easier. You can also try a very small amount (check with your pediatrician for dosage) of milk of magnesia every day until the problem resolves. Rectal stimulation is another tried and true remedy. Use a rectal thermometer dipped in some KY Jelly (not petroleum jelly), and move it gently in and out of the rectum. This stimulation will usually produce a stool, but you may want to be ready for it to come out quickly!

Babies, before they walk, are much like bedridden adults. Constipation is a common problem in adults in nursing homes. So, it makes sense that more stagnant babies are constipated, too. Older people can get obsessed with their bowel habits. You never see a constipated athlete, though, do you? Once the baby is walking, moving, and shaking, stooling usually becomes an everyday thing. They're also eating things like hotdogs and vegetables, which make for a much different stool. Breastmilk is so bioavailable (readily utilized by your baby's body) that there isn't really much waste.

Diarrhea Should Not Be Taken Loosely

Most breastmilk stools are loose. This is to say they're very liquidy, like diarrhea. This is a good thing and nothing to call the pediatrician about. Again, breastmilk is a perfect food and results in lots of stools during the day. These stools are usually relatively small and do not have much of a smell to them. If your baby is having multiple large, liquidy "blowouts" per day, possibly associated with pain, then call your pediatrician's office.

A Note on Diaper Cream

Think about it—babies poop and pee in their diapers all day long. Regardless of how absorbent diapers are, feces and urine will still be touching the skin at some point. For this reason, you should apply a good layer of some brand of zinc oxide ointment on the skin. It's the same stuff lifeguards used on their noses back when your mother was a kid—that white stuff that's so hard to wipe off. Remember to put it on clean, dry skin. If you're changing wet diapers and you've applied enough butt paste previously (like you're spackling in drywall), all you have to do is put a new diaper on the baby. Another benefit of zinc oxide is that if there's only a little bit of poop, you can feed first and hold off on rushing to the changing table. This is helpful because you can count on another poopy diaper almost every time the baby eats!

I'm not a big fan of either diaper wipes (don't like the chemicals) or rubbing baby's tender skin. You've heard the expression "soft as a baby's bottom?" Well, that soft skin is tender and you need to be gentle. If you're cleaning a poopy diaper, especially on a newborn with a diaper rash, I usually put baby under a high faucet (I implore you to **check** the water temperature first) and let the water pressure do the work. Use Cetaphil or another gentle cleanser to clean the baby's tushie. You can also use a small, baby washcloth. When dry, spackle in the drywall (so to speak) with diaper cream.

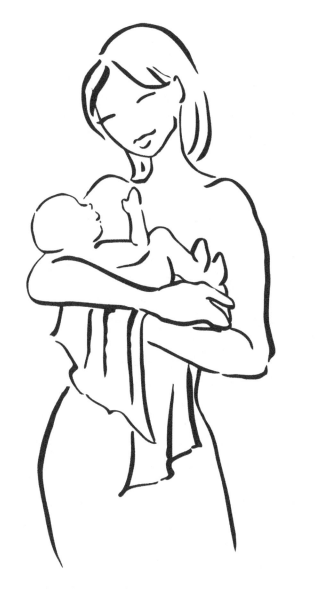

Part III

FROM THE WORLD OF THE LACTATION CONSULTANT

Chapter 10

Real Questions by Real Mothers and Real Answers by a Real Lactation Consultant

Question: *Help! My baby won't nurse for even five minutes, and all she does is cry. What am I doing wrong?*

My daughter has never sucked for long at my breast. She cries, I put her to the boob, and she mostly doesn't do much. You say that you should hear the babies move from "suck suck suck swallow, suck suck suck swallow" in the initial 1-2 minutes to "suck swallow, suck swallow" once your MER (milk ejection reflex) takes over and your breasts produce milk. This never happens for me. I can't get her to do a "suck swallow."

Answer: If your baby is gaining weight, then five minutes may be enough. If she's gaining an extraordinary amount of weight, then perhaps your letdown is too strong, and she can't organize her suck swallow because of the pressure, and that's causing her to cry.

You won't always hear your baby swallow in the first week. Try hand expressing your milk onto the tip of your nipple prior to latching her onto the breast. Then you know it's there and you've "primed the pump." You can continue with some breast compressions during the feed, which will help get her started. Be calm and patient. If all else fails, try the "basket of rolls" trick: Give her a bit of breastmilk by bottle, cup, or syringe, and then bring her back to the breast.

If your baby is not gaining weight, I'd encourage you to find a lactation consultant as soon as possible, but in the meantime, get busy maintaining your supply with a good quality hospital grade breastpump.

Question: *What are the initial warning signs that I should look for to indicate that I am not producing enough milk? What can I do about this problem at an early stage?*

Answer: It is important to recognize the initial signs, so you can attack the problems early. Some initial warning signs are:

- You are unable to hand express any colostrum.
- You don't hear a "suck swallow, suck swallow" pattern of eating.

- Your baby does not have any or many wet and poopy diapers.

- Your baby is not gaining at least one ounce of weight per day.

- Your baby has no moisture in his mouth, and/or your baby has urate crystals (looks like brick dust) in his diaper.

If you can't hand express anything and your baby is crying when you bring him to the breast, try a hospital-grade pump. If a hospital-grade pump is not helping, contact a lactation consultant to watch an entire feeding. The lactation consultant can help you do a pre- and post-feed weight to see how much the baby received.

Question: *How aggressive should I be in trying to get my baby to suckle?*

Answer: When you put your baby to your breast, you don't need to be forceful. You can tickle his feet, undress him, or tap on his chin to get him awake and interested. Lots of skin-to-skin contact is always helpful. Count to 10 by one-Mississippi, two-Mississippi, etc., and if he hasn't begun sucking again on his own by the count of 10 (not two, three, or five), you can nudge him, preferably on his feet or shoulder. You should minimally be able to get at least 30-60 seconds of nursing at a time. If you find yourself needing to forcefully molest your baby to get him to nurse, use the pump and bottle-feed some of that feeding. If you don't have enough milk, try some formula (½ - 1 oz), and then try him back at the breast an hour later.

Question: *My baby has jaundice and the feedings take FOREVER! (Sometimes more than 45 minutes on one breast). I feel like all I do is feed her, and the feedings seem a lot longer than all the books say they should be. Is this normal? Will I ever be able to do anything but nurse?*

Answer: Just remember, your priorities should simply be to stimulate the milk and feed your baby. Don't torture yourself or your baby. You can start to make your own schedule, as there are no other hard and fast rules. As one mother lamented to me, you are never going to look like the mother on the baby book cover, and that is okay.

Yes, I know most books state that your baby will typically feed for 10-30 minutes. However, in reality, there actually is a much wider range of normal for nursing. It's not a particularly bad thing for your baby to nurse for a long period of time once in awhile, but you can't possibly keep up that schedule all day every day. An entire nursing/feeding session shouldn't really take more than 40 minutes, start to finish. However, there are a lot of factors to consider, including: your baby's weight, if your milk supply is established, if you're supplementing, what your nipples feel like, and whether or not you're pumping.

Question: *How do I know when my baby is DONE feeding and not just taking a quick break?*

Sometimes my baby comes off my breast after eating for 20 minutes. I burp him and offer the other breast, but my baby won't take it. When I think the feeding is over, I start my 20 minutes of pumping. Fifteen minutes into pumping, though, my baby starts screaming. I know he wants more food, but I had just pumped for 15 minutes AFTER feeding him, so I thought putting him BACK to the breast seems futile because there wouldn't be anything there.

Answer: Initially, your baby's messages to you may seem inconsistent and confusing. It will take a bit of time to learn your baby's eating habits. It could be that he is not sure what he wants. Even I will sneak back into the kitchen to steal a cookie after I've eaten a huge meal. Try to discern whether it happens all the time or once in awhile? If it happens all the time, and you don't want to keep putting your baby on and off your breast, then I recommend you stop pumping when your baby starts to scream (whether it's five minutes or 15 minutes), and put him to the breast. Alternatively, you can feed any milk you've pumped to your baby, and then see if he is more satisfied. Remember that your breasts are never empty! Even if you've just pumped for 20 minutes, I guarantee you that there's still some milk in the breasts. You can put baby on at ANY time.

If your son clenches his fists after you feed him, it may indicate he is still hungry. After getting some food, his hands will probably open like blooming flowers, and you should get the "Weekend at Bernies" effect. Read the section "Ensuring Baby Eats When Hungry" in Chapter 1 on inborn feeding cues to help you understand what hungry might look like.

Question: *I want to breastfeed my child, but I don't seem to have enough supply, even if I pump and breastfeed frequently (all day long actually). I don't want to introduce formula because I know it will just reduce my supply more, but it pains me to see my child screaming because he is hungry. What do I do?*

Answer: You have to walk a narrow line between what you're trying to do to exclusively breastfeed and having a hungry baby. You need to really check if the baby is getting what he needs. You can rent a baby scale, so you can ensure your baby is gaining weight. Unfortunately, the scales for sale at the local baby store are not accurate enough. Renting is always a better option in this instance. There's nothing wrong with trying some comforting techniques, but if they're not working, you can absolutely feed the baby a little bit of formula. Although this can be a slippery slope, it can also be the thing that saves the breastfeeding relationship.

Question: *Is it normal for babies to want to snack every hour all day long? I can't keep up with the constant eating. What should I do?*

Answer: Yes, it's common (and OK) for babies to eat like little hummingbirds all day long. They are using your breasts as vessels for feeding, but also as a source for comfort and support, as they explore their world throughout their day. The question is, "Is it OK with YOU?" If it is, then go right ahead. Your comfort is important, too. If constant feeding is not working for you, try some other calming techniques to make it to the next feeding. Your baby is not getting enough to eat if the calming techniques are not working, there aren't at least six to eight wet diapers a day (after the fifth day), or your baby is NOT gaining weight.

Question: *I can't get the baby to latch properly. I've tried what the books say to do, namely opening up my daughter's mouth to a "full upright and locked position" and "rubbing my nipple on her upper lip, expressing some milk and rubbing that on her lips, etc." I still end up with incredibly sore nipples. What should I do now?*

Answer: Find yourself a good lactation consultant to help you with this one. In the meantime, keep trying to get her to latch. Pump both breasts at least every 2½-3 hours during the day, and every three to four hours at night for a full 20 to 30 minutes. After trying to get baby to latch, go ahead and feed the pumped milk with a good orthodontic nipple. That way, by the time you and the consultant meet, you'll at least have maintained your milk supply and have a satisfied baby.

Question: *Should I be putting the baby to my breast every two to three hours during the day, despite her utter disinterest in nursing and her desire to sleep?*

Answer: This answer partially depends on the age of your baby. If it's during the first 14 days and your baby is not gaining at least one ounce per day, then yes, keep putting your baby to your breast and nurse her. If your baby is gaining one or more ounces per day, then you can take breaks of 2½ - 3 hours. Make sure there are some excellent feeding sessions, meaning that your breasts are noticeably softer after feeding and your baby looks and acts satisfied. Also, read "Sleeping with Baby" in Chapter 5. You may want to wake her during the day, so you're not up the entire night. Having said this, if your baby is gaining adequately, you're enjoying the schedule, and it works for you, there is no one right way to schedule her.

Question: *Is it really true that you need to "get nursing established for three or four weeks before introducing a bottle, so the baby won't refuse the breast?"*

Answer: Yes, that would be preferable, but with one caveat. If your baby is jaundiced, then there is a medical reason to use the bottle and nipple early on. This trumps the perfect sucking that comes with waiting to use a bottle.

What you DON'T want is your baby to prefer the easy, quick flow of a rubber nipple in his mouth. All that does is raise his expectations for how much food is to be delivered at a feeding. If you have a perfectly healthy baby, you don't need to wait until your baby is well established at the breast before using lots (more than two a day) of bottles. One or two relief bottles a day (filled with your milk) should not cause a problem. It usually only takes babies a week or two before they're well established, but it could take longer.

Question: *I heard that if I don't feed my baby with a bottle early on, she will never learn to use one. Is this true?*

Answer: Yes, there is a window within the early months in which you should start giving your baby a bottle or two a day. This is especially important for mothers who are going back to work. When your baby gets used to breastfeeding, she gets all the love, warmth, closeness, and attention from you by using her reflexive sucking action. Further down the road, her sucking becomes a voluntary action, and she can become more fickle about what she will suck. It's as if your baby is thinking, "Hmmm, maybe I'll suck and maybe I won't...mom will have to ask herself whether she feels lucky."

Chapter 11

Questions I've Been Asked and Other Unbelievable Tales I Couldn't Possibly Have Made Up!

Look Who's Talking Now

You may want to talk to your baby ALL DAY LONG. They love the sound of your voice, and it makes them feel comforted. In order to model appropriate parenting techniques, I talk to the babies when I'm examining them. "OK, now I'm going to look into your ears, I'll be really quick, and then..." You get the idea. One day, during my exam, as I'm bent over the baby, I feel a tap on my shoulder and the dad proclaims, "Excuse me Kathy...errrrrrrr, he doesn't understand you." WHAT??? I couldn't believe it. I guess we shouldn't talk to them for a few years then!

No More Dog-Breath

If it's not one thing, it's your mother. My (s)mother was staying with us one weekend to "help" me with the kids while my husband was away on a business trip. She came into the kitchen for breakfast and remarked that we had the worst tasting toothpaste she'd ever tasted. Asking what flavor it was, I remarked that it was our dog's *chicken-flavored* toothpaste. Perhaps one needs to put their glasses on prior to brushing one's teeth in the morning? My kids and I laughed and laughed and laughed.

The Perils of Multi-Tasking

It's easy to understand why mothers need to multi-task; we have a bazillion things to do. I wonder how sleep deprived one particular mother was when she asked me if she could take her sitz bath and pump her breasts at the same time. I'm pretty sure electrocution might have been a real possibility had she gone through with it.

Sibling Rivalry

A few months after bringing my second baby home from the hospital, I noticed my 22-month-old son pushing the baby's bassinet towards the down-staircase. As he was pushing, he put together his first sentence, "Baby OUT." Umm, there were certainly no subtleties in that message. Of course, my daughter had her justifiable revenge when her first big word was "Adam-did-it."

I've heard people say that bringing a new baby home is analogous to your husband bringing home a new wife (which I might not have minded if she would have shared the workload back then, but I digress). Keep in mind this is a difficult time for the reigning king or queen at home. Make some special mommy and daddy time to soften the blow. Also remember, they don't want a lot of gifts, they want YOU.

Keep in mind that when you're home alone with two kids, you're no longer playing man-on-man, you're now playing ZONE DEFENSE.

Adventures of Supermom

When my first baby, Adam, was born, I can remember doing (or trying to do) everything perfectly. I was going to be a superhero mom and make sure nothing hurt my baby. One day, while strolling down my street, I even grabbed a bee in mid-air because I thought it was flying too close to Adam's stroller. Things in my home could not possibly be clean enough, bottles couldn't be sterile enough, and people couldn't possibly be healthy enough to hold or touch Adam (I still stand by this last one). Anyway, fast-forward to when my daughter was about a year old and I find her on her knees, barking, and eating out of the dog bowl. All I remember saying to myself is, "Huh, that's clean kibble in that bowl." See the difference? Just to note that in my own personal longitudinal study, both kids turned out to be great, healthy adults, regardless of exposure to germs!

Choosing a Nickname

I worked with a lovely first-generation Japanese family who came to my office and announced that even though their son had a proper, formal, first name, they were going to call him *Nookie*. Whoa, I just couldn't let that happen and told them what *other* meaning that word had here in the U.S. The father couldn't seem to bow enough during that visit when he said to me, "Ohhhhh thank you, Kathy-San, you've saved my first son much embarrassment in his life. We will change his nickname."

To My Days With My Own Babies

As your kids get older, you'll welcome the joys and challenges from them that are very different and yet almost eerily similar to the challenges you now face with your infant.

I suffered severe sleep deprivation when my babies became teenagers, and then when they started to drive. It was reminiscent of having a newborn, in that you keep waking up just to check that they're still breathing. I would wake up and look at the clock wondering if they were home safely yet, then I'd have to tip-toe to their room and see if I slept past them sneaking into the house.

Both of my kids are in their mid-twenties. I feel like they are happy, thriving adults, so I'm thinking the hardest part is over. Now that they're both out of the house, though, I find myself using an Urban Dictionary to get through a conversation with them. I sit at my computer and wait to type in a word they use, so I don't seem as dumb as they might think. I remember my son telling me he was a *Baller.* I gasped and told him I hoped he was "using protection," until my comment was met with raucous laughter telling me that's *Not what he meant...* If you don't know what this means, you need to look it up, too! Very enlightening, I tell you.

There's also a big difference between male and female adult children. They both say the same thing, but in very different ways. Adam comes home and wants to know what kind of beer I have. Erin comes home and informs me that, "Nobody wears that color eye shadow anymore." I do enjoy having a daughter, though, just for that reason. She also let me know that she thought my underwear was "way too big," and we immediately embarked on a trip to Victoria's Secret. The bottom line (no pun intended) is that I think she attempts to keep me young. (Notice I say *attempts* here?) Considering she's the one that gave me the grayest hair, I'd say that's only fair.

Hopefully, by now you've learned new ways to navigate through and enjoy this new experience that seems to defy your endurance, and yet somehow doesn't. Remember, some day your kids will be teenagers, and you'll have a whole new set of challenges and joys!

American Academy of Pediatrics Task Force on Sudden Infant Death Syndrome. (2005). The changing concept of sudden infant death syndrome: Diagnostic coding shifts, controversies regarding the sleeping environment, and new variables to consider in reducing the risk. *Pediatrics, 116*(5): 1245-1255.

Academy of Breastfeeding Medicine. (2007). ABM Clinical Protocol #2 (2007 revision): Guidelines for hospital discharge of the breastfeeding term newborn and mother: "the going home protocol." *Breastfeeding Medicine, 2*(3), 158-165.

BFHI. (1991). Handling and storage of breastmilk. Retrieved on 11/19/10 from http://www.aap.org/breastfeeding/faqsBreastfeeding.html.

Blumenthal, J. A., Babyak, M. A., Doraiswamy, P. M., Watkins, L., Hoffman, B. M., Barbour, K. A., et al. (2007). Exercise and pharmacotherapy in the treatment of major depressive disorder. Psychosomatic Medicine, 69(7), 587-596.

CDC. (2010). Proper handling and storage of human milk. Retrieved on 11/19/10 from www.cdc.gov/breastfeeding/recommendations/handling_breastmilk.htm.

Cobo, E. (1993). Characteristics of the spontaneous milk ejecting activity occurring during human lactation. *Journal of Perinatal Medicine, 21*(1), 77-85.

Colson, S. (2008) *Biological nurturing: Laid-back breastfeeding.* Hythe, Kent, UK: The Nurturing Project.

Colson, S. (2003). Cuddles, biological nurturing, exclusive breastfeeding and public health. *Journal of the Royal Society of Health, 123*(2), 76-77.

Cotterman, K. J. (2004) Reverse pressure softening: A simple tool to prepare areola for easier latching during engorgement. *Journal of Human Lactation, 20*(2), 227-237.

De Carvalho, M., Robertson, S., Friedman, A., Klaus, M. (1983). Effect of frequent breastfeeding on early milk production and infant weight gain. *Pediatrics, 72*(3), 307-311.

Dewey, K. G., & McCrory, M. A. (1994). Effects of dieting and physical activity on pregnancy and lactation. *American Journal of Clinical Nutrition, 59*(2 Suppl), 446S-452S; discussion 452S-453S.

Eidelman, A. I., Hoffmann, N. W., & Kaitz, M. (1993). Cognitive deficits in women after childbirth. *Obstetrics and Gynecology, 81* (5 (Pt 1)), 764-767.

Geddes, D. T., Kent, J. C., Mitoulas, L. R., & Hartmann, P. E. (2008). Tongue movement and intra-oral vacuum in breastfeeding infants. *Early Human Development, 84*(7), 471-477.

Genna, C. W. (2008). Breastfeeding: Normal sucking and swallowing. In C. W. Genna

(Ed.), *Supporting sucking skills in breastfeeding infants* (pp. 1-41). Boston, MA: Jones and Bartlett.

Glover, R., & Wiessinger, D. (2008). The infant-mother breastfeeding conversation: Helping when they lose the thread. In C. W. Genna, (Ed.), *Supporting sucking skills in breastfeeding infants* (pp. 97-129). Boston, MA: Jones and Bartlett.

Hale, T. W. (2010). *Medications and mother's milk* (14th ed.). Amarillo, TX: Hale Publishing.

InfantRisk Center. (2010). Alcohol and breastfeeding. Retrieved on 11/19/10 from http://infantrisk.org/category/alcohol.

Ingram, J. C., Woolridge, M. W., Greenwood, R. J., & McGrath, L. (1999). Maternal predictors of early breast milk output. *Acta Paediatrica, 88*(5), 493-499.

Karp, H. (2003). The happiest baby on the block – The new way to calm crying and help your baby sleep longer (DVD). The Happiest Baby, Inc.

Kendall-Tackett, K. A. (2005). *The hidden feelings of motherhood: Coping with stress, depression, and burnout.* 2nd ed. Amarillo, TX: Pharmasoft Publishing.

Kendall-Tackett, K. (2007). A new paradigm for depression in new mothers: The central role of inflammation and how breastfeeding and anti-inflammatory treatments protect maternal mental health. *International Breastfeeding Journal, 2,* 6.

Kendall-Tackett, K. (2009). *Postpartum depression at a glance.* Amarillo, TX: Hale Publishing.

Kendall-Tackett, K. (2010). *Depression in new mothers: Causes, consequences, and treatment alternatives* (2nd ed.). New York, NY: Routledge.

Kent, J. C., Mitoulas, L. R., Cregan, M. D., Geddes, D. T., Larsson, M., Doherty, D. A., et al. (2008). Importance of vacuum for breastmilk expression. *Breastfeeding Medicine, 3*(1), 11-19.

Kemp, C. (October, 2005). Preventing SIDS: AAP task force updates recommendations to reduce risk of sudden infant death syndrome. *AAP News, 26,* 1-12.

La Leche League International. (2010). What are the LLLI guidelines for storing my milk? Retrieved on 11/19/10 from http://www.llli.org/FAQ/milkstorage.

Medela. (2010). Nipple shields. Retrieved on 11/19/10 from http://www.medelabreastfeedingus.com/tips-and-solutions/112/nipple-shields.

Mohrbacher, N. (2010). *Breastfeeding answers made simple: A guide for helping mothers.* Amarillo, TX: Hale Publishing.

Mohrbacher, N., & Kendall-Tackett, K. (2010). *Breastfeeding made simple: Seven natural laws for nursing mothers.* 2nd ed. New Harbinger Publications: Oakland, CA.

National Conference of State Legislatures. (2010). Breastfeeding state laws. Retrieved on 11/19/10 from www.ncsl.org/IssuesResearch/Health/BreastfeedingLaws/tabid/14389/Default.aspx.

Neville, M. C., Keller, R., Seacat, J., Lutes, V., Neifert, M., Casey, C., et al. (1988). Studies in human lactation: milk volumes in lactating women during the onset of lactation and full lactation. *American Journal of Clinical Nutrition, 48*(6), 1375-1386.

Neville, M. C., Allen, J. C., Archer, P. C., Casey, C. E., Seacat, J., Keller, R. P., et al. (1991). Studies in human lactation: Milk volume and nutrient composition during weaning and lactogenesis. *American Journal of Clinical Nutrition, 54*(1), 81-92.

Newman, J. (2010). Candida protocol. Retrieved 11/19/10 from http://www.drjacknewman.com/help/Candida-Protocol.asp.

Prime, D. K., Geddes, D. T., & Hartmann, P. E. (2007). Oxytocin: Milk ejection and maternal-infant well-being. In T. W. Hale & P. E. Hartmann (Eds.), *Hale & Hartmann's Textbook of Human Lactation* (pp. 141-155). Amarillo, TX: Hale Publishing.

Ramsay, D. T., Kent, J. C., Owens, R. A., & Hartmann, P. E. (2005). Anatomy of the lactating human breast redefined with ultrasound imaging. *Journal of Anatomy*, 206(6), 525-534.

Ramsay, D. T., Kent, J. C., Owens, R. A., & Hartmann, P. E. (2004). Ultrasound imaging of milk ejection in the breast of lactating women. *Pediatrics*, 113(2), 361-367.

Simple Wishes. (2010). Hands free pumping bra. Retrieved December 8, 2010, from http://www.simplewishes.com/.

St. James-Roberts, I., Bowyer, J., Varghese, S., & Sawdon, J. (1994). Infant crying patterns in Manali and London. *Child: Care, Health and Development, 20*, 323–337.

Top 25 Grandparent Quotations – Claudette Colbert. Retrieved October 10, 2010, from http://ezinearticles.com/?Top-25-Grandparent-Quotations&id=14161.

West. D., & Marasco, L. (2009). *The breastfeeding mother's guide to making more milk*. New York, NY: McGraw Hill.

Widstrom, A. M., Ransjo-Arvidson, A. B., Christensson, K., Matthiesen, A. S., Winberg, J., & Uvnas-Moberg, K. (1987). Gastric suction in healthy newborn infants. Effects on circulation and developing feeding behaviour. *Acta Paediatrica Scandinavica, 76*(4), 566-572.

Wright, K. S., Quinn, T. J., & Carey, G. B. (2002). Infant acceptance of breast milk after maternal exercise. *Pediatrics, 109*(4), 585-589.

Alcohol – Whiskey, wine, beer, and other fun ways to relax you.....just take it EASY.

Baby Blues – A common, temporary state of mood swings, irritability, depression, anxiety, and crying that occurs after childbirth. Any woman that has experienced PMS totally gets it.

Baby Friendly Hospital Initiative – Launched in 1991 by UNICEF and WHO to insure that all hospital and maternity facilities (birthing centers) support breastfeeding using specific parameters and steps. Bottom line is, if the hospital is designated as "baby friendly," they won't try to give you and your baby formula and other things that undermine mom's breast intentions (pun intended).

Bilirubin - The end product of red blood cell destruction. It's what turns babies into Aztec suntan gods and goddesses.

Block Feeding - A feeding pattern for over-supply issues whereby a mom uses one breast for a specific "block" of time. It helps to calm down the (.)(.) girls.

Breast Compression - Compressing the breast to ensure adequate drainage while you're breastfeeding.

Breast Sandwich – The lovely oval shape one needs to smush the breast into when trying to put a decent amount of breast tissue into the little bird mouth.

C-Hold – Holding the fingers around the breast to resemble the letter C.

C-Section – Surgery through the abdomen to ensure a healthy baby and mom.

Cluster Feed – Baby feeds, feeds again an hour later, and then feeds one more time until you think you can't take it anymore. Then, just when you think they've got to be full, they feed again......you get the point!

Colic – Cranky, crying, at times inconsolable, fussy babies have "colic."

Colic-Hold – A hold illustrated in the text to help babies get a grip. In this hold, gentle pressure is placed on the left side to help aid digestion and burping, making baby more comfortable.

Cradle Hold – Holding the baby in the classic hold that you see on infant product brochures. You make a cradle out of both arms at once, with no holding of the breast.

Cross Cradle Hold – The opposite from the cradle hold. If the baby is latching onto the left breast, you hold the left breast in your left hand and the baby's head in your right, with baby across your body.
Football Hold – Baby tucked under your armpit, with the opposite side hand supporting your breast, and the same side hand supporting baby's head.

Foremilk – Satisfies thirst; the first milk, higher in lactose, that is expelled from the breast when moms start to breastfeed or pump. (See hindmilk for what comes next).

Frenulum – Specifically, the lingual frenulum, meaning the string under the tongue that may or may not be too tight. When too tight, babies need to dart their tongues in and out "a la lizard" to get any milk. OUCH!

Gastroesophageal Reflux Disease (GERD) – When the muscle that connects the esophagus (food tube) to the top of the stomach allows milk to reflux back up and produce a burny, acidy, painful feeling that turns babies into Oscar the Grouch (rightfully so…remember what that felt like when you were pregnant, mom?).

Hindmilk – Comes after foremilk and satisfies appetite. This milk is richer and higher in fat.

Jaundice - Yellowing of the skin and whites of the eyes when there is too much bilirubin in the body. It turns babies into "Weekend at Bernie's." If you haven't seen the movie, think dead tired.

Kegels – What you would have to do with your va-jay-jay to stop urine mid-stream if someone opened the bathroom stall door, and you had to get up and close it.

Labia – The outside lips of your vagina.

Letdown – When the showerhead (nipples) starts sprinkling milk out. Technically, we call it a milk ejection reflex. The nipple sends the message to your pituitary to send a message to the breast to "let 'er rip." It will happen one to four times during the course of a nursing or pumping session.

Linea Negra – The black vertical line from your rib cage or belly button to your pubic hair that you're worried won't go away (but usually does and probably will).

Lochia – Postpartum vaginal discharge containing blood, mucus, and uterine tissue that hangs around like a period for a month or longer.

Mastitis – A breast infection causing pain, chills, inflammation, redness, malaise, and flu-like symptoms.

Milk Ejection Reflex - When your milk starts to flow out the nipple pores after a short time of baby's suckling. This is also called your letdown or letdown reflex.

Nadir Weight – The lowest weight your baby ever reaches, usually on day two or three postpartum.

Nipple Shield – Looks like a silicone sombrero for a mouse. Gives your baby something to latch onto when you have flat or inverted nipples.

Obligate Nose Breathers – All babies ONLY breathe out of the noses until they're about four to six months old. Boogers can cause a lot of problems during this time.

Pacifier – That little rubber thing resembling a nipple that parents think babies need constantly. Personally, I think it's more for the parents than for the babies.

Plugged Duct – An area of the breast where milk flow is obstructed. This lump usually develops slowly and only affects one breast, causing localized pain, but rarely systemic symptoms. Get help early, so it doesn't turn into mastitis.

Postpartum Depression – A prolonged feeling of sadness and depression more severe then baby blues.

Primary Engorgement – When your milk first comes in and you wake up looking like a porn star.

Probiotic – The opposite of an antibiotic. A product that builds bacteria instead of destroying it. Think live yogurt cultures multiplied in pill or powdered form.

Reclining Position – Mom lies back on pillows to relax and lets gravity hold her baby to her body.

Respiratory Syncytial Virus – A mean, ugly virus that can wreak havoc with baby's respiratory system. To be avoided at all costs.

Reverse Pressure Softening – A method of softening the areola without removing milk.

Side Lying Position– Lying on your side to breastfeed baby.

Sling – A piece of cloth used to hold baby against you, allowing your hands to be free.

Stool Guaiac Test – A test to determine whether or not there's blood in the stool.

Suck Spot – An area on the roof of the mouth that, when pressure is applied, causes reflexive sucking.

Swaddling (also called bundling) - A way of turning baby into a papoose, using a blanket, to elicit sleep or to calm baby. It blunts feeding cues, so take it easy here.

Tail of Spence - Breast tissue located all the way up and into the armpits. This tissue can swell dramatically when milk comes in, causing you to look like a line backer.

Tummy Feeding – Baby on top of your tummy during a feeding.

Tummy Time – Baby laying flat on the his stomach to give him time to practice head lifting and to ensure he doesn't end up with a head that's flat like a pancake from spending all day and all night on his back.

Umbilical Granuloma – A piece of living tissue that remains after the belly button stump falls off. To seal over the skin, this area may need to be cauterized with a silver nitrate stick. This is the same way a veterinarian will stop bleeding on your dog's paws when he snips a bit too much nail off.

Warrior Skills – When you put on your big girl panties and suck it up to help you get to where you want to be with breastfeeding.

Web Sites for Additional Information

- www.aap.org/breastfeeding
- www.cdc.gov/breastfeeding
- www.drjacknewman.com
- www.infantrisk.org
- www.kellymom.com
- www.lowmilsupply.org
- www.llli.org
- www.mobimotherhood.org
- www.mother-food.com
- www.ncsl.org/IssuesResearch/Health/BreastfeedingLaws/tabid/14389/Default.aspx/

Products Mentioned

- Breastfeeding Pillow - www.BethesdaBreastfeeding.com
- Simple Wishes Bustier (hands-free pumping bra) - www.simplewishes.com
- Soothies - www.lansinoh.com/products/soothies-by-lansinoh-gel-pads

Recommended Breastfeeding Books

The Nursing Mother's Companion by Kathleen Huggins (Harvard Common Press; 6th edition; 2010)

The Ultimate Breastfeeding Book of Answers by Dr. Jack Newman and Teresa Pitman (Three Rivers Press; revised edition; 2006)

The Womanly Art of Breastfeeding by Diana Wiessinger for La Leche League International (Ballantine Books; 8th revised edition; 2010)

Kathleen F. McCue, MS, RN, FNP-BC, IBCLC, is both a nurse practitioner and a board-certified lactation consultant. She is the mother of two grown children and currently lives in Bethesda, MD. She has been working in the medical field since 1976 when she first graduated nursing school. Presently, she works part-time as a nurse practitioner for a pediatric practice, Children First Pediatrics, and part-time operating a full-service lactation consulting business, Bethesda Breastfeeding, LLC, in the Washington, D.C. area.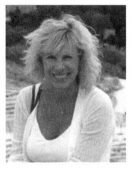

Kathleen's first exposure to breastfeeding and its benefits came nearly 20 years ago when she was working as a nurse in a local pediatric practice. She saw that breastfeeding offered a wide range of health advantages, but it had little public recognition and acceptance. Working with breastfeeding mothers and babies offered Kathleen a great deal of personal satisfaction. In 2000, Kathleen returned to school for her Nurse Practitioner degree, and chose Family Practice as her specialty. NP training brought new information and insight that Kathleen immediately put to good use with new mothers. At the same time, her expanded experience and confidence helped bring greater reassurance and calm to women seeking to breastfeed for the first time.

Although breastfeeding outcomes and infant health issues are serious, Kathleen has found that new mothers benefit from understanding they are not alone and from hearing about innumerable other women who have faced the same issues. She uses the humor of shared human experience to help new moms cope. There will always be another situation or predicament that is more unusual, more unique, or otherwise just able to make a mom under stress lighten up and laugh. With humor, Kathleen helps put new moms at ease, while constantly reassuring them that breastfeeding can and will work, and that relaxing can actually facilitate the process.

Kathleen wanted to write this book to give new parents an easy-to-read reference—and she just could not say "yes" to everyone who asked if she "could please come home with us." She hopes readers will be more informed and reassured after reading this book, and that it will make the breastfeeding process easier and less stressful. Nothing should be more natural. Her website can be found at www.bethesdabreastfeeding.com.

70712540R10080

Made in the USA
Middletown, DE
28 September 2019